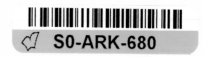
S0-ARK-680

AGING IN THE NEW MILLENNIUM

Social Problems and Social Issues
Leon Ginsberg, Series Editor

To the memory of my cousins who did not have the opportunity to be old—Anna Hernandez, age 57 years; Rita De Palma, age 60 years; Jean Dossiano, age 56 years; Ignacio Palermo, age 55 years; Russell Palermo, age 52 years—and to their surviving sister, Minnie Mendola, who is a courageous ager

depression, Alzheimer's disease, alcoholism and drug abuse, and anxiety disorders.

Chapter Eight presents myths, stereotypes, and research on the attitudes of both young persons and the elderly about the aging process. The material also includes attitudes of professionals about working with older adults and the attitudes about aging in other countries.

Chapter Nine discusses the experiences of aging for women, gay men and lesbians, and ethnic groups.

Chapter Ten focuses on programs and services for older persons including an overview of major public-support programs and home care, hospice, adult day care, nursing homes, respite care and recreation, nutrition, housing, elder abuse, education, and intergenerational programs. Case examples are included.

Chapter Eleven outlines the impact of the longevity explosion on political, social, and economic systems.

Chapter Twelve concludes with a discussion of emerging future and unresolved issues such as longevity versus quality of life, public-policy choices versus private choices, interdependence or intergenerational conflict, spirituality and religion, assisted suicide and the right to die, and a proposal for courageous aging. Research studies, statistics, current knowledge, and future trends are presented to provide the reader with current and essential information regarding concepts, theories, and issues in aging. Internet sites, books, and journals are suggested for further study of selected topics. It is the author's hope that learning about aging will inspire courageous aging and will promote future interest in gerontological research.

ACKNOWLEDGMENTS

I would like to thank the special people who were so important to me in writing this book. Leon Ginsberg encouraged me to take on the project. Frank Raymond III, dean of the College of Social Work at the University of South Carolina, provided me with much-needed support. My research assistants, Holly Kaufman, Marilyn Jackson, Lindsay Spradley, and Jeounghee Kim, were quite dedicated. They spent many hours searching for material and working tirelessly, even on weekends, researching materials for this book. I would like to thank Carlos Torres for his research on global aging and Angela Alfano for her fastidious editing, which brought the manuscript to its present state. I especially appreciate the generosity of my colleagues who shared family pictures with me. My son, Dr. Sal Tirrito, shared his medical knowledge with me and answered my many questions. My daughter Catherine and her family, Mike, Michael, and Nicholas, reminded me of the future. Finally, I would like to thank my husband, Sal, for believing in and encouraging my dreams.

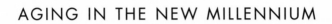

AGING IN THE NEW MILLENNIUM

CHAPTER ONE

Global Aging

> . . . in recognition of humanity's demographic coming of age, the promise it holds for maturing attitudes and capabilities in social, economic, cultural and spiritual undertakings, not least for global peace and development in the next century.
>
> UNDPI 1996, 1

To mark the end of a century that saw unprecedented growth worldwide, the United Nations General Assembly designated 1999 as the International Year of Older Persons. The extraordinary growth of the aging population in almost every country in the world is referred to as *global aging*. Aging in the new millennium will be very different from aging in the twentieth century.

In the twentieth century, reduction in infant mortality, improvements in health status, and new medical technologies contributed to longer life expectancy, increasing the number of persons surviving into old age. Although life expectancy increased universally, life expectancy in developing countries is still lower than in developed countries. Gender differences are found in life expectancy and in health worldwide. Nations are struggling with the social and economic impacts of global aging with respect to changes in dependency ratios, pension reforms, health care, and rising costs for long-term care. The social and economic results of the growth of the general population, infant mortality rates, and fertility rates influence the longevity and quality of life of the older population.

The world population in 1945 was 2.3 billion. It is predicted to increase from 5.4 billion people in 1995 to 9.4 billion by 2050. Annual growth is estimated at 81 million. Eighty percent of the world population (4.3 billion) lives in underdeveloped countries, while 1.1 billion live in the more developed areas (UNPD-DESIPA 1997).

The general population is anticipated to grow in Africa and Asia with minimum growth in Europe and North America. Africa's greatest population growth rate occurred from 1950 through 1995 (271%, or about 2.6% per year). The Latin American/Caribbean population soared from 166 million persons to 477 million, or a growth of about 2.3% per year. Asia's population consecutively mounted by about 2% per year, while Europe's population increased by about 0.6% per year. Western Europe had the highest annual growth rate as a result of in-migration. Eastern Europe had negative population growth caused by out-migration, decline in fertility, and rising mortality rates. Both Southern and Northern Europe experienced a decline in population growth due to a decrease in fertility rates. Fertility rates are an important factor in the longevity equation. In countries where more children are born and other factors are conducive, it can be expected that more people will live to old age.

According to a United Nations Population Division study (1995), for the following regions the total fertility rate per 100 births is

Africa	5.7 births
Latin America/Caribbean	2.9 births
Asia	2.8 births
North America	2.0 births
Europe	
Lowest total fertility rate: Italy	1.2 births
Highest total fertility rate: Albania	2.9 births

Total fertility rates, infant mortality rates (per 1,000 live births), civil wars, migrations, and diseases are factors that affect population changes and affect the longevity rate. Africa and Asia experienced the largest population growth. By 2050, 79.9% of the world's population will be living in these two regions. Latin American/Caribbean populations, likewise, demonstrate a pattern of continuous growth. North America and Oceania appear to be undergoing moderate growth. European trends indicate that there will be a continuing population decline in the coming decades from 21.7% of the world's population in 1950 to 6.8% in 2050 (UNPD-DESA 1998).

Table 1.1 Africa's Regions

Eastern	Middle	Northern	Southern	Western
Burundi	Central African Republic	Algeria	Angola	Benin
Comoros		Egypt	Botswana	Burkina Faso
Djibouti	Chad	Libya	Lesotho	
Eritrea	Congo	Morocco	Madagascar	Cameroon
Ethiopia	Equatorial Guinea	Sahara	Malawi	Cape Verde
Kenya		Sudan	Mozambique	
Mauritius	Gabon	Tunisia	Namibia	Côte d'Ivoire
Reunion	Republic of the Congo (formerly Zaire)		South Africa	Gambia
Rwanda			Swaziland	Ghana
Seychelles			Zambia	Guinea
Somalia	San Tome & Principe		Zimbabwe	Guinea-Bissau
Tanzania				
Uganda				Liberia
				Mali
				Mauritania
				Niger
				Nigeria
				Senegal
				Sierra Leone
				Togo

Source: United Nations Publications, 1996

An influencing factor, particularly in the next century, is the infant mortality rate. Children must survive to reach adulthood. The average global infant mortality rate is 62 deaths per 1,000 live births. Government efforts to further reduce infant mortality rates, if successful, will categorically increase life expectancies. The average global life expectancy in 1997 was 65 years, and in 2045 it is expected to reach 76 years (Chamie 1997).

Table 1.2 Regional Infant Mortality Rate: Africa (per 1,000)

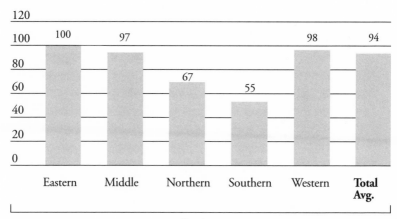

Region

Source: UNPD-DESIPA, 1997

Africa

Statistics for regional infant mortality and fertility rates in Africa are presented in tables 1.1, 1.2, and 1.3.

Africa has regions that differ widely in general population growth, fertility rates, and infant mortality rates, and these regions will differ in life expectancy rates. The Northern and Southern regions of Africa have the lowest infant mortality rates. The Middle region has the next lowest, followed by the Western and Eastern regions at 100 per 1,000 births. The regions with the highest infant mortality rate also have the highest fertility rates, with the Eastern region being the highest. The Northern and Southern regions are quite similar, with fertility rates of 4.1 and 4.2 per 100, respectively (UNPD-DESIPA 1997).

While Africa's population reached 224 million in 1950, statistical data reveal that in 1995 its population more than tripled in size to 720 million. As of 2050, the population is expected to reach 2.1 billion (Heilig 1996). Africa has the lowest life expectancy of all seven regions of the world; three of its countries have the lowest of all world populations (UNPD-DESIPA 1997). Low life expectancy rates, high fertility rates, and high infant mortality rates are predicted to continue in Africa if economic and political conditions remain unchanged.

Table 1.3 Regional Fertility Rate: Africa (per 100)

Bar chart showing fertility rates by region: Eastern 6.4, Middle 6.4, Northern 4.1, Southern 4.2, Western 6.4, Total Avg. 5.7. Y-axis from 0 to 7. X-axis labeled "Region".

Source: UNPD-DESIPA, 1997

Table 1.4 Asia's Regions

Eastern	South Central	South Eastern	Western
China	Afghanistan	Brunei	Armenia
Democratic People's Republic of Korea	Bangladesh	Darussalam	Azerbaijan
	Bhutan	Cambodia	Bahrain
Japan	India	Indonesia	Cypress
Mongolia	Iran (Islamic Republic of)	Lao (People's Democratic Republic)	Georgia
Republic of Korea	Kazakhstan		Iraq
	Kyrgystan	Malaysia	Israel
	Maldives	Myanmar	Jordan
	Nepal	Philippines	Kuwait
	Pakistan	Singapore	Lebanon
	Sri Lanka	Thailand	Oman
	Tajikistan	Vietnam	Qatar
			Saudi Arabia
			Syria Arab Republic
			Turkey
			United Arab Emirates
			Yemen

Source: United Nations Publications, 1996

Table 1.5 Regional Infant Mortality Rate: Asia (per 1,000)

	Eastern	South Central	South Eastern	Western	**Total Avg.**
Value	41	78	54	60	62

Region

Source: UNPD-DESIPA, 1997

Table 1.6 Regional Fertility Rate: Asia (per 100)

	Eastern	South Central	South Eastern	Western	**Total Avg.**
Value	1.9	3.7	3.2	4.1	2.8

Region

Source: UNPD-DESIPA, 1997

Asia

Asia contains more than half the world's inhabitants. In 1950, Asia had 1.4 billion people. Asia's population reached a total of 3.4 billion people in 1995. Projections are that the population will climb to 5.4 billion people by the year 2050 (Heilig 1996). The low total fertility rate in Eastern Asia is partly due to China's one-child-per-family policy. South Central Asia's total fertility rate is one reason that India will surpass China in total population in the future. Statistics show that Eastern Asia has the lowest fertility rate. South Eastern and South Central Asia follow with fertility rates of 3.2 and 3.7 per 100, respectively. Western Asia follows with the highest fertility rate, at 4.1 per 100. Infant mortality rates are highest in South Central Asia, averaging 78 births per 1,000. Western, South Eastern, and Eastern Asia are moderately lower.

Table 1.7 Latin American/Caribbean Regions

Caribbean	Central America	South America
Antigua and Barbuda	Belize	Argentina
Aruba	Costa Rica	Bolivia
Bahamas	El Salvador	Brazil
Barbados	Guatemala	Chile
Cayman Islands	Honduras	Colombia
Cuba	Mexico	Ecuador
Curaçao	Nicaragua	Guyana
Dominica	Panama	Paraguay
Dominican Republic		Peru
Grenada		Suriname
Haiti		Uruguay
Jamaica		Venezuela
Saint Vincent & the Grenadines		
Saint Kitts and Nevis		
St. Lucia		
Trinidad & Tobago		

Source: UNPD-DESIPA, 1997

Table 1.8 Regional Infant Mortality Rate: Latin America/
Caribbean (per 1,000)

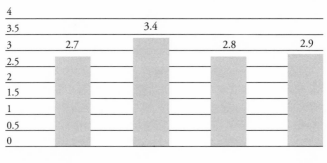

	Caribbean	Central America	South America	**Total Avg.**
	43	37	41	40

Region

Source: UNPD-DESIPA, 1997

Table 1.9 Regional Fertility Rate: Latin America/Caribbean
(per 100)

	Caribbean	Central America	South America	**Total Avg.**
	2.7	3.4	2.8	2.9

Region

Source: UNPD-DESIPA, 1997

Latin America/Caribbean

The Latin American/Caribbean regions grew from 166 million people in 1950 to 244 million people in 1995 and are expected to reach 810 million by 2050 (Heilig 1996). Statistics for regional fertility rates and infant mortality rates are presented in the tables 1.7, 1.8, and 1.9.

Infant mortality rates are highest in the Caribbean and lowest in Central America, with South America falling in between with 41 per 1,000 births. Fertility rates seem to be highest in Central America, followed by South America and the Caribbean (UNPD-DESIPA 1997).

Europe

Europe's population rose from 547 million (1950) to 728 million (1995) and is expected to decrease to 595 million by 2150 (Heilig 1996). A low fertility rate is one reason why Europe's population is decreasing. In contrast to other world regions, Europe's fertility rates

Table 1.10 Europe's Regions

Eastern	Western	Northern	Southern
Belarus	Austria	Denmark	Albania
Bulgaria	Belgium	Estonia	Andorra
Czech Republic	France	Finland	Bosnia-Herzegovina
Hungary	Germany	Iceland	
Moldova (Republic of)	Liechtenstein	Ireland	Croatia
	Luxembourg	Latvia	Greece
Poland	Monaco	Lithuania	Holy See
Romania	Netherlands	Norway	Italy
Russia Federation	Switzerland	Sweden	Macedonia (Former Yugoslav Republic of)
Slovakia		United Kingdom	
Ukraine			Malta
			Portugal
			San Marino
			Slovenia
			Spain
			Yugoslavia

Source: United Nations Publications, 1996

Table 1.11 Regional Infant Mortality Rate: Europe (per 1,000)

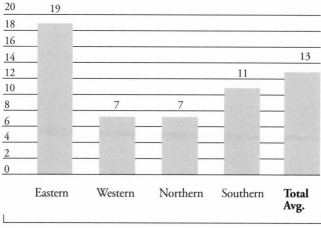

| | Eastern | Western | Northern | Southern | **Total Avg.** |

Region

Source: UNPD-DESIPA, 1997

Table 1.12 Regional Fertility Rate: Europe (per 100)

| | Eastern | Western | Northern | Southern | **Total Avg.** |

Region

Source: UNPD-DESIPA, 1997

are among the lowest in the world, falling between 1.4 (Southern Europe) and 1.8 per 100 births (Northern Europe) (UNPD-DESIPA 1997).

North America and Oceania

An increase in in-migration has caused North America to experience stimulated growth. Since 1950, North America's population rose from 172 million people to 297 million people. The anticipation is that total population will reach 384 million people by the year 2050 (Heilig 1996).

Oceania is composed of Australia/New Zealand, Melanesia, Micronesia, and Polynesia. Oceania's population has evolved from 13 million (1950) to 28 million (1995), and will expand to 46 million by the year 2050 (Heilig 1996). The total fertility rate of Australia/New Zealand is 1.9%, while the infant mortality rate is 7 births per 1,000 and life expectancy is 77.4 years (UNPD-DESIPA 1997). The changes in population growth will impact the lives of older persons worldwide.

Growth of Aging Population

Some countries categorize people ages 65 years and above as being old. Some countries use 60 years of age as the marker for old age. In this book, data are reported for both ages. Commonly used terms to identify aging groups are the young-old (65–74 years), the old (75–85 years), the old-old (85–90 years), and the very old (90+ years). The old-old are the fastest growing and most vulnerable group (Johnson and Barer 1997).

The extraordinary growth rate in the aging population globally is a result of a decline in death rates in all age groups, major reductions in infectious and parasitic diseases, decreases in infant and maternal mortality rates, and improvements in nutrition, health services, education, and income. Birth rates and death rates determine population aging. Populations age as fertility rates decline and mortality rates improve.

The world's older adult population (older than 60 years) will grow from one-half billion in 1990 to 1.5 billion in 2050 (UNDPI 1996). Between 1995 and 2150, this group is expected to expand from 9% to 30% of the world's total population (UNDP-DESA 1998).

By the middle of the twenty-first century, the percentage of those persons 60 years and older will be greater than those 15 years and

Table 1.13 The World's Old-Old

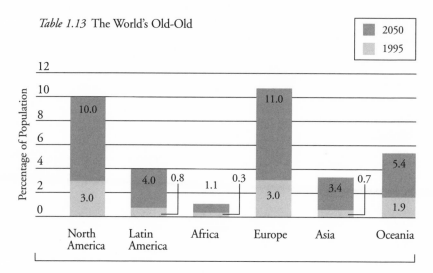

Region

Source: Koster and Prather, 1997

younger. The percentage of those persons 80 years and older will increase substantially. By 2025, 72% of the world's older adult population will live in Africa, Asia, Latin America/Caribbean, parts of Europe, and Oceania (UNDPI 1996). China and the region of Latin America/Caribbean are facing a doubling of the proportion of their older adult population.

The world's elderly population is increasing at the rate of 800,000 persons each month. With the current incremental monthly gain, projections for the year 2010 indicate consecutive monthly net gains of 1.1 million. The growth rate of the elderly population in developing countries is two times that of the world's population of all ages.

Europe is the oldest world region and Africa is the youngest. Europe's 65 years and older population is 14% of its total population. By the year 2025, more than one in ten Europeans will be 75 years or older. Both North America and Oceania's elder population is expected to increase dramatically. Growth in Asia and Latin America is likewise predicted to increase significantly (U.S. Bureau of the Census 1992).

Gender differences exist in the growth of the older population. In Italy in 1990, there were two older women (older than 80 years) for each man. In Italy, the population of older persons older than 60 years is expected to grow from its current portion of 19.8% of the population to 21% by 2020. In 1950, the population older than 60 was 12.2%.

The dependency ratio of the older-than-80 group is a concern as the population of persons younger than 20 years of age decreases. In the early part of the century, 15 to 17 million persons in Italy were younger than 20 years of age. The number younger than 20 years of age is predicted to be less than 9 million in 2020 while the older-than-80 group is expected to be 3.2 million in 2020, or 6.1% of the population older than 60 years of age. This change in the young-old ratio will have a profound effect on the social and health-care systems of that country (Lori et al. 1999). This trend is common among other European countries.

Developed and developing nations are discovering that the 80 years and older age group is the fastest-growing population in the elderly, a phenomenon without historical precedent. The old-old constituted 16% of the world's elderly in 1992 (22% in developed countries and 12% in developing countries). In France, Germany, and Sweden, 25% of the elderly population is 80 years and older. Forty percent of the old-old reside in three countries: China, the United States, and the former Soviet Union. In 1990, the percentages of the old-old ranged from 0.2% in Indonesia and Kenya to 4.4% in Sweden. In each nation, the 85 and older population is predominately female.

In 1998, the United Nations began the process of gathering population statistics for the purpose of estimating and predicting age groups 80–84, 85–89, 90–94, 95–99, and 100 and older. In Canada, 350,000 persons ages 85 and older accounted for 1.2% of the population. Projections are that this age group will continue to increase until 2041, when it will represent 4% of Canada's population. In a remote area of Bama, China, there are more than 280 people older than age 90. Researchers have investigated diet, air quality, climate, environment, and the absence of pollutants to explain this unusual phenomenon. By 2050, the old-old will constitute 7.4% of the population in North America, 4.0% in Latin America and the Caribbean, 1.1% in Africa, 7.9% in Europe, 3.4% in Asia, and 5.4% in Oceania (Koster and Prather 1997).

Dependency Ratio

The *dependency ratio,* or number or proportion of individuals in the dependent segment of the population divided by the number or proportion of individuals in the working population, determines the support of older persons by younger persons in each country. The dependency ratio has two segments: the old and the young, or the old (65 and older) and the working (18 to 64). The old age dependency ratio is calculated as 65+ / 18–64 x 100. Table 1.14 is an example of dependency ratios in the United States.

As shown in table 1.14, the ratio suggests that in the year 2000 every 21 individuals older than 65 will require support from 100 working persons (ages 18 to 64 years). In the years 2010 and 2020, when the baby boomers reach retirement age, the number of persons who will be supported by working persons will increase substantially, and in 2040, every 37 persons older than 65 will be supported by 100 working persons.

The Berlin Aging Study examined 500 Germans whose ages ranged from 70 to 100 years. This study is reported to be one of the world's largest interdisciplinary studies of the old-old. The study found

Table 1.14 Old Age Dependency Ratios, 1970 to 2050 (U.S.)

Year	Ratio
1970	17.6
1980	18.6
1990	20.2
2000	20.9
2010	21.5
2020	27.4
2030	35.7
2040	37.1
2050	36.2

Source: U.S. Bureau of the Census, 1995

evidence of intergenerational sharing in this age group whereby older adults helped their friends, families, and neighbors by providing child care, taking care of vacationing relatives' pets, preparing meals, helping homebound elders, doing yard work, and making repairs. This study concludes that dependency will not be a social burden.

More than four million Americans were 85 years old in 2000, and by 2030, 8 million are expected to reach this plateau. Another international study found that the amount of assistance given to the old-old in the United States was extremely low when compared to the amount of assistance provided by European nations to their old-old. In America, the old-old are often left alone, with help provided by public-service programs. Among older Americans, 30% did not receive from agencies or organizations the type of assistance they required to perform basic daily tasks, compared to 1% of Swedes. The level of care provided by formal agencies drops as Americans age. Almost four in ten Americans ages 85 or older report having unmet needs such as bathing, dressing, using the toilet, preparing meals, or doing housework. Older people who reported needing assistance in these areas stated that assistance was not received. The old-old, the most vulnerable of the aging population, is the group that receives the least assistance (Jarrott et al. 1998).

A significant proportion of the world's older persons live in rural areas. Africa, Asia, and Latin America/Caribbean can anticipate their

Table 1.15 Rural Elderly by World Region

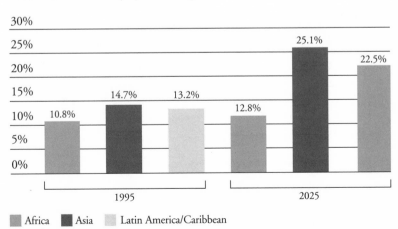

Source: http://ftp.fao.org/waicent/faoinfo/sustdev/wpdirect/wpan0016.htm (1998)

rural elderly population will almost double from 215 million people to almost 400 million people between 1995 and 2025. The rural elderly dependency ratio (the proportion of the 60 and older population to that of those 15 to 59 years of age) will likewise increase in these regions (du Guerny 1997).

The World's Oldest Countries

Although some countries have higher numbers of older persons in the general population, until recently Sweden had been considered the world's oldest country because 18% of its population is composed of older persons. However, in 1996, Italy and Greece moved ahead with the largest percentage of older people in the world (more than 22%). In most countries older populations ranged between 16% to 22% of the general population. If the former Soviet Union had remained intact, it would have been fourth in world status with 28 million older persons, following China, India, and the United States. More than 15 million of all elderly persons in the former Soviet Union live in Russia and one-fourth of these are concentrated in the Ukraine. Russia's elderly population is expected to double in size by the year 2025. Traditionally, Islamic countries have experienced declines in fertility since the late 1950s.

Globally, the median age is expected to rise. The median age divides a population into numerically equal parts of younger and older persons. The median age in Kenya is 15 years and in Sweden it is 39 years. In Kenya, the number of people younger than 15 years of age is equal to the number older than 15 years of age. It is projected that in 2025 Italy will have the highest median age with nearly half of its population ages 50 and older as a result of an extremely low fertility rate. The median age in the world population will rise from 25.4 years in 1995 to 36.5 years in 2050 (U.S. Bureau of the Census 1992). The contrast in median age between Sweden and Kenya illustrates the differences in population aging in developed and developing countries.

Social and Economic Impact of Global Aging

Africa, Asia, and Latin America can anticipate a doubling of the elderly population between 1995 and 2025. Asia and Latin America can expect to see tremendous growth in the rural elderly dependency ratio,

Table 1.16 The World's Oldest Countries: Percentage of Population Age 60 and Older

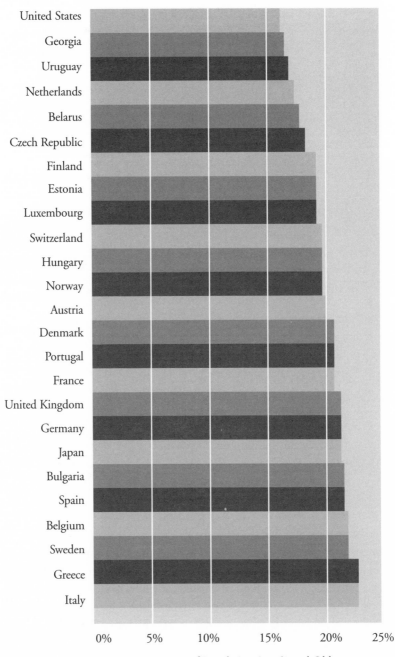

Percentage of Population Age 60 and Older

Source: UNPD—DESIPA

from 15% to 59%, as younger adults leave rural areas for jobs in urban areas and older persons are left behind. By 2025, there will be about 50 million older adults in Africa and 337 million in Asia (du Guerny 1997).

Social and economic concerns include health services, pensions, social supports, land and property ownership, and inheritance issues. In the United States, Canada, Australia, New Zealand, and Europe, economic security for older women; rising costs of health-care services; growth of age-specific institutions; access to educational, cultural, spiritual, and recreational resources; employment of older persons; and living environments must be addressed. How will governments prepare?

Challenges and questions are unanswered and unresolved. Decisions and answers will be needed to resolve these questions. For example, what should governments and other private and/or not-for-profit agencies do to prepare to provide older adults with the tools necessary to maintain independence and dignity? The United Nations encourages governments to address these issues:

* Fostering independence
* Encouraging participation in community life and politics
* Ensuring accessibility to care services to maintain physical, emotional, and mental health
* Ensuring accessibility to resources to nurture self-fulfillment
* Creating financial environments that encourage people to save for their old age
* Strengthening measures and mechanisms to ensure that retired persons do not fall into debt and poverty
* Encouraging and supporting cross-generational participation in policy and program development and in decision-making bodies at all levels
(UNDPI 1996)

Non-governmental organizations (NGOs) are joining local governments and governmental agencies to meet these objectives. An example of a non-government agency is HelpAge International, a reputable worldwide network of not-for-profit organizations. Its mission is to work with and for disadvantaged older adults to improve the quality of their lives (HelpAge International 1997). HelpAge has different programs in each country.

❖ **Cambodia**: There are programs for resettlement and reintegration of older refugees, providing loans to assist older Cambodians to become self-sufficient, setting up and improving eyecare services (cataract surgery), and participating in the National Committee for the Prevention of Blindness.

❖ **Sri Lanka**: In conjunction with Sri Lanka Scout Association, HelpAge provides material care and moral support to elderly refugees.

❖ **Singapore**: HelpAge works with Tsao Foundation (founded in 1993 by 94-year-old Mrs. Tsao Ng Yu Shun as a family foundation) to improve the lives of older adults by providing:
  • Community Health Services—a continuum of services using the case manager primary care model.
    a) Hua Mei Mobile Clinic—medical and health care for home-bound elderly
    b) Hua Mei Seniors Clinic—outpatient geriatric care
    c) Hua Mei Acupuncture Clinic
  • Training and Education—disseminating information and providing training to caregivers, the elderly, and health-care providers.
  • Interagency Collaboration—promoting resource sharing, networking of agencies, and international exchanges of information.

❖ **Pakistan:** HelpAge collaborates with Pakistan Medico International to provide "eye camps" offering needed cataract surgery, glasses, and medications for eye infections.

❖ **Korea**: HelpAge established Help Home Services in 1987 to help elderly with household work, bathing, laundry, cooking, and transportation.
  • In 1997, Home Help Services joined Seoul Municipality and forty-eight other organizations to form the Korea Association of Community Care for the Aged to help the elderly maintain independent lives in the community.
  • A Day Care Center Program provides protection and help at home.
  • A Job Placement Service was begun in 1992 with Seoul Municipality to provide vocational training, orientation, and job-placement services for the working elderly.

❖ **Thailand**: HelpAge supported the Klong Toey Slum Project, which provides comprehensive health care and facilitates net working.
  • In 1996 and 1997, it provided basic living supplies to Burmese refugees in Mae Sot (Thai-Burmese border).
  • In 1997, it worked with the British Embassy to fund a Day Care Center for Older Akha People (in Northern Thailand) providing health care and financial support (i.e., older adults passing on traditions like Akha weaving and crafts to younger people), health checks, and education.
  • It collaborated with Women Against AIDS to form "Support for Older People Affected by HIV/AIDS Programme."
  • The Asia Training Centre on Aging (ATCOA), founded in 1992 by HelpAge International, reaches twenty-two countries in Asian/Pacific areas offering training workshops and consultation services (New Age Asia staff 1996).

❖ **Macao**: Instituto de Acao Social de Macao (Department of Social Welfare of the government of Macao) provides discount cards to older citizens for clothing, food, transportation, and medical treatment (New Age Asia staff 1996).

❖ **Fiji**: HelpAge Fiji opened a gift store selling items made by older people.

❖ **Ghana**: HelpAge Ghana is working with Aseseeso Age-Care Society to form a community farm. This farm helps to provide a better diet for older adults.

❖ **Uganda**: The Anglican Church offers residential placement and assists older persons to build their own homes (Nkoyoyo 1995).

❖ **Bolivia**: HelpAge works with Centre de Investigacion y Promocion Education in assisting older people in the Altiplano region to turn hostile, arid land into crop-producing (green vegetables, potatoes) farms.

❖ **St. Lucia**: In 1993, HelpAge St. Lucia worked with the St. Lucia Blind Welfare Association to form "Club 60" programs, a network of social and welfare clubs for older adults and, in 1995, helped to establish the National Council of and for Older Persons to build network relations of all age organizations on St. Lucia.

❖ **Europe**: HelpAge works with nineteen other organizations in twelve countries to foster the networking and sharing of information and resources among older adults.

Economic and Political Stability

Governments must provide economic and political stability for their citizens. The reallocation of resources and services now distributed to the younger population is essential as the population ages (Beattie 1995). Beattie suggests that governments could gradually increase the pension age by generating more jobs, especially for women and older adults. Paul and Paul (1995) advocate the implementation of an international social security tax to help fund social programs around the world, a change which would mean a major shift in people's conception from national to global planning. Governments are re-examining their pension systems and looking for reforms and new systems to ensure economic security for older adults.

The United Nations advocates that it is safer and wiser for individuals to save for their own old age. In 1993, 14 million pensioners received an average of U.S. $132 per month, with minimum necessities costing U.S. $327 a month. Table 1.17 presents an overview of the disparity between actual pension amounts and the cost of basic essentials in some South American countries.

The Chilean Model of Pension Reform

The Chilean Model of Pension Reform is an example of pension reconstruction. Chilean reformation requires all employers to reduce an employee's earnings by 10% and to deposit these deductions into annuities operated by companies called Administradora de Fondos de Pensiones (AFP). Neither employers nor governments need contribute any additional amounts nor bear any other responsibility except for a weak "safety net" program for the elderly poor.

In addition to the 10% deduction from each employee's earnings toward their pensions, the AFP deducts 2% from the worker's gross pay for administration fees and 1% for disability insurance. Additionally, workers pay a minimum of 7% of their gross pay (depending on the level of coverage) for health insurance (Fazio and Riesco 1997). A total

Table 1.17 Pensions in Selected South American Countries

Country	Monthly Pension Amount (in US $)	Cost of Necessities
Bolivia	78	307
Colombia	123	400
Peru	90	250
Venezuela	90	183
Argentina	300	1,085

Source: Adapted from http://www.globalaging.org/resource/pubs/jpaul.htm, 1994

deduction of 20% (10 + 1 + 2 + 7) is taken out of the employee's gross pay. This system has been in place in Chile since 1981, and it is mandatory that all new employees participate in the AFP system. Pre-reform employees, although free to continue in the old pension system, were strongly urged by the AFP companies and the government to switch to the new system. "The main incentive was that under the new system (AFP) employers' contributions are directly added to gross pay and had the effect of raising the gross pay by 30%" (Fazio and Riesco 1997, 90). Accordingly, if pre-reform employees had switched to the new system, their gross pay should have increased by 10% (30%–20%).

A pension system that encourages people to save for the future and fosters independence is a logical concept. However, the questions of how much one is required to earn and what measure of time one needs to work in order for the system to function are not yet resolved. In addition, the pension system in Chile does not report favorable results for all employees. Paul and Paul (1995) found inequities regarding pension reform in the case of military officers and privileged social groups because their pensions were not reduced—nor were the pensions of lower-paid workers increased—with the AFP system. Accounts that have more to invest grow faster. Since the government no longer contributes to the pension system, it utilizes this "savings" to underwrite debts owed by private Chilean banks to foreign lenders, thereby protecting the investments of a few wealthy banking families.

The "safety net" comes to about U.S. $36 per month, about enough to buy a loaf of bread and a cup of coffee each day. Additionally, there is a maximum limit of 300,000 older adults eligible to receive this safety net.

In addition, the AFP does not adequately administer the redistribution of pensions. Strong supplemental social insurance for the unemployed, disabled, or others who experience a loss of income (whether temporary or long term) resulting in lower pensions is nonexistent. Pre-reform retirees, who are in the old system, must depend on the government's making the right decision in regard to pension allotments. The current retiree allowance is about U.S. $66 per month. International analysts have predicted that, under the Reformed Chilean System, at least half of all retired workers' benefits will fall below the poverty level (Diaz 1995).

The World Bank is working diligently for government adoption of pension reform in Africa and Asia. In China, family and collectives have been the traditional supports for the elderly. Collectives are government sponsored and guarantee housing, food, medical care, clothing, and funeral costs (Paul and Paul 1995). Because unemployment rates have increased, families are less able to provide on their own for older family members, and older workers are encouraged to take early retirement to make room for younger workers (Paul and Paul 1995).

The World Bank, International Labour Organization, World Health Organization, United Nations Development Program, universities, and private consulting firms are initiating solutions to pension reformation. Two models have been proposed. One is a social-security model; the other is modeled after that of the Chilean Reform Pension System and is favored by the World Bank and supported by the State Commission of the Economic System (Cooper 1998).

Nkoyoyo (1995) reported that international monetary lenders encouraged the government in Uganda to adopt reform policies (i.e., Adjustment Program) by scaling down the number of workers. In developing nations, pension reforms are a major concern for governments. Government institutions in both Europe and North America are considering the restructuring of existing pension systems. Due to the high cost of reunification, the German government is considering cuts in its pension system. Presently, men receive DM 1,600 a month (about U.S. $1,000) and women receive DM 900 a month (about U.S. $600).

However, for many pensioners their only income source is the pension. Companies are increasingly switching to a part-time labor force to limit their responsibilities to provide benefits to employees (LaFontaine 1997). Paul and Paul (1995) reported that Sweden and Italy are considering cutting back on pension benefits. In the United States, the U.S. Congress is considering social-security reforms such as privatizing the social-security program. Great Britain has instituted a semi-privatization process of pensions. Sweden and Italy are looking at similar plans (Paul 1995).

In a comparative study of national policies for aged care and support, Kane (1998) reported differences in the United States, Australia, Canada, and Germany. All four countries provide for retirement and assure that all retirees are covered with at least a minimal pension. The United States and Germany have more universal programs while Canada and Australia rely on individual retirement programs. All four countries provide some type of universal health insurance for older persons. In the United States, health insurance coverage is provided for those older than 65 years by Medicare if the individual contributed to the Social Security system, or by Medicaid, a state means-tested program for the poor. In the other three countries health insurance is universal.

There are many differences in the four countries in the approach to long-term care. The Canadian system has broad and generous long-term-care coverage for institutional and community care. While long-term care is free, some provinces require the residents of nursing homes to pay a co-payment to cover room and board. The American system relies on the state-funded Medicaid program, a means-tested welfare program operated by states with matching federal funds. Most states have eligibility requirements for state residents that require a spend-down of their assets to become eligible.

The Australian system has a mixed state and federal system in which federal programs pay for institutional care and require co-payment for the cost of room and board. State and federal governments pay for the cost of community care. Germany pays for all institutional care and provides a pension and stipend for caregivers. There is opportunity to receive cash in lieu of services, and about half of nursing home residents receive social-aid welfare. In the United States, Canada, and Australia, the area of emphasis in long-term care is first the institution, then the community. In Germany the emphasis is community and then institution (Kane 1998). The assurance of health services to an aging population demands that governments recognize the importance of psychological, social, cultural, and environmental influences. Globalization—what takes place in one world region—likewise affects other regions. Economic stability will impact the lives of older persons around the world.

Social Supports

Changes are expected in family supports in both developing and developed countries. Traditionally, families have been the key supports for older adults in most countries. Older adults provide support to families in the care of grandchildren, passing on cultural and family customs while passing on land and wealth. The emergence of the "nuclear family" in developing countries has created new situations for older persons in the traditional family. Conversely, in developed countries the disintegration of the nuclear family has altered what was formerly considered the "traditional family." The composition of the nuclear family is usually two parents and their children.

While the concept of the nuclear family is held as the ideal family image in the United States and other developed nations, this is not the typical family in other parts of the world. The growth in non-nuclear-type families is negatively interpreted as a result of the breakup of the traditional family unit, which previously included grandparents and extended family members (Nkoyoyo 1995). Many families in developing regions have limited financial means, and pensions of older adults in the home often supplement the family income. Strong economies have contributed to the changes in family structures, with the younger person earning income freedom to live separately from parents. In addition, older persons with pension security have income freedom to live independently.

World population planning reports for the United Nations promote reduction of fertility rates, particularly in heavily populated nations. China's one-child-per-family policy is an example. However, in countries

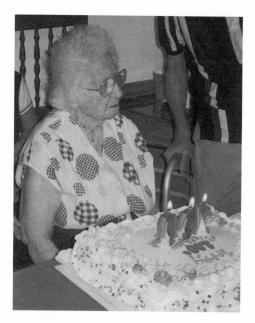

Eightieth birthdays and one hundredth birthdays are more common today than they were in the past.

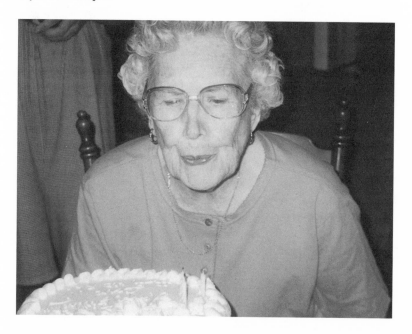

where reduction in fertility rates is encouraged, will older adults receive help (Paul and Paul 1995)? The "one child's" resources will be further stretched as she or he cares for two parents. As life expectancy increases, the "one child" will probably have the extra burden of also caring for grandparents. Without some level of government-supported income, families will not be motivated to stabilize or decrease the fertility rate, thus placing additional stress on population development plans (Paul and Paul 1995).

Globally, women face special challenges as they grow older. Traditional roles for older women consist of caring for grandchildren, households, and communities. In Nigeria, older women are childbirth attendants, and in China, domestic work by older women allows younger women to take a greater role in the labor force (Sadik 1996). Women are less likely to have a significant work history (a recognized, paid one), more likely to have lower-paying jobs, and more likely to have less total time and smaller amounts of money to put into a retirement account. In some countries, women are not allowed to own land or to have inheritance rights. Women are more likely to be poorer in old age than men (Miller 1999). Because women live to older ages than do men, they are at greater risk for experiencing chronic health problems and social and economic deprivation.

Political Stability

In some regions of the world, civil wars have claimed millions of lives and have caused massive displacement of the region's inhabitants. In the latter part of 1995, 5.7 million people were exiled in Africa (1.3 million in Zaire and 0.7 million in the United Republic of Tanzania). One million of Somalia's citizens sought refuge in other areas as a result of its crisis; one-quarter of these people have returned (UNPD-DESIPA 1997). The Sudan admitted many refugees and became a springboard for about 350,000 people who advanced to the Central African Republic, Ethiopia, Kenya, and Zaire. In 1995, 1.1 million Rwandan citizens fled to Zaire and another 0.5 million escaped to the United Republic of Tanzania. Civil strife in Liberia resulted in 300,000 persons seeking refuge in Côte d'Ivoire while 400,000 sought refuge in Guinea (UNPD-DESIPA 1997). Rwanda and Togo also have experienced outflows of their populations.

In Asia, the South Central area is home to a large concentration of refugees, about 16 million people. These refugees are survivors of the 1948 partitioning of India and the invasion of Afghanistan by the former Union of Soviet Socialist Republics during the 1980s. Cambodia has experienced two decades of civil wars from the1970s through the 1980s (HelpAge International 1997).

Persons seeking refuge inside the former Yugoslavian borders in mid-1984 escalated to 3.8 million (2.7 million in Bosnia-Herzegovina and 0.5 million in Croatia). By the end of 1995, there were still 1.3 million displaced persons in former Yugoslavia (1.1 million residing in Bosnia-Herzegovina). Since the end of the Cold War, some Eastern European countries and the former Union of Soviet Socialist Republics have relaxed their exit regulations. This policy created an increase in migration to Western Europe among the younger generations. Almost 24 million refugees immigrated to North America, 20 million of whom relocated to the United States (UNPD-DESIPA 1997).

Civil wars catastrophically affect elderly people. The aftermath of a civil war may result in the loss of home and country, family supports, and sometimes the added burden of caring for orphaned grandchildren. The demise of younger family members and sudden displacement from their homelands intensifies the older adults' daily struggle for support systems.

Health Issues

Health issues that primarily affect younger adults can also impact the lives of older persons. As of 1995, Africa had 70% of the world's HIV/AIDS cases while Asia had 6% (UNPD-DESIPA 1997). The Population Division Department for Economic and Social Information and Policy Analysis of the United Nations Secretariat listed twenty-eight countries in which either about 2% of the adult population is currently infected with HIV or the absolute number of infected adults is very high.

In some African countries, India, Thailand, Brazil, and Haiti, AIDS is having the effect of lowering a country's life expectancy by six years. India and Thailand are expected to have substantial increases in the rate of new infections, surpassing even the rate of infections in Africa. Between 1995 and 2015, Asia's share in total number of AIDS-related deaths will rise from 3% to 47%. How does this devastating situation affect the older adult population? The older population often must provide care for those affected and are often the ones left behind without the support of their children. Most cases of HIV/AIDS infections and deaths are found in persons between ages 20 and 59 years. Their deaths and failing health necessitates that the older adult family members care for them and their grandchildren (Dennerstein et al. 1998).

Summary

Aging in the new millennium will vary among different areas of the world. Developed countries can expect increases in life expectancy with increases in populations of rural older persons and dependency may be a problem for Europe and North America, but quality-of-life issues and economic security will take precedence for most governments. Pension reformation and reorganization of government policies are essential for the coming century.

References

Beattie, R. 1995. *Pensions and pension reform.* Presented at the World Summit on Social Development, March, Copenhagen, Denmark. On-line: http://www. globalaging.org/resources/copenhagen/bettie.htm

Chamie, J. 1997. *Statements to the Commission on Population and Develop-ment (thirteenth session).* Speech presented to the meeting of the United Nations Commission on Population and Development, February, United Nations, New York.

Cooper, M. 1998. Chile's pension mirage. Excerpts from article in *The Nation* (Mar.): 12, 16, 20. On-line: http://www.globalaging.org/pension/world/ chile2.htm

Dennerstein, L., S. Feldman, C. Murdaugh, J. Rossouw, and S. Tennstedt. 1998. Gender and health issues in aging. In *1997 World Congress of Gerontology, Aging Beyond 2000: One World One Future*, supplement to *The Australiasian Journal on Aging* 17 (1): 19–21.

Diaz, A. 1995. *The pension crisis in Argentina.* World Summit on Social Develop-ment, March, Copenhagen, Denmark. Global Action on Aging. On-line: http://www.globalaging.org/resources/copenhagen/diaz.htm

du Guerny, J. 1997. *The rural elderly and the aging of rural population.* Presented at the World Congress of Gerontology/Inter-Agency Meeting for the International Year of Older Persons 1999, August, Adelaide, Australia. On-line: http:// ftp.fao.org/waicent/faoinfo/sustdev/Wpdirect/Wpan0016.htm

Fazio, H., and M. Riesco. 1997. The Chilean pension fund associations. *New Left Review* 223 (May/June): 90–100. On-line: http://www.globalaging.org/ pension/world/chilepen.htm

Heilig, G. 1996. World population prospects: Analyzing the 1996 UN Population Projections. Unpublished manuscript. On-line: http://www.iiasa.ac.at/ Publications/Documents/WP96–146.html/frmain.htm

HelpAge International. 1997. *Aging in Asia and the Pacific and what we do.* On-line: http://chmai.loxinfo.co.th/helpage/Aging_in_Asia/SRILANKA.htm

Jarrott, S. E., S. H. Zarit, S. Berg, and L. Johansson. 1998. Adult day care for dementia: A comparison of programs in Sweden and the United States. *Journal of Cross Cultural Gerontology* 13 (2): 99–108.

Johnson, C. L., and B. Barer. 1997. *Life beyond 85 years: The aura of survivorship.* New York: Springer Publishing.

Kane, Robert. 1998. Comparative national policies on care and support of older persons. In *1997 World Congress of Gerontology, Aging Beyond 2000: One World One Future*, supplement to *The Australiasian Journal on Aging* 17 (1): 42–46.

Koster, J., and J. Prather, eds. 1997. Counting the world's oldest citizens. *Global Aging Report* 2 (1) (Jan./Feb.): 5.

LaFontaine, O. 1997. *The future of German social democracy.* Excerpts from a speech to the SPD Conference, December, Hanover, Germany. On-line: http://www.globalaging.org/pension/world/lafontai.htm.

Lori, A., A. Golini, B. Cantalini, P. Bruno, F. Citoni, and F. Paganelli. 1999. *Prinicipali risultati.* On-line: http://www.aging.cnr.it/atlante.htm.

Miller, Claudia. 1999. The oldest Americans: Resilient but having to struggle. *Aging Today* 20 (1) (Jan./Feb.): 14.

New Age Asia staff. 1996. *Asia Regional Newsletter,* no. 4 (June). On-line: http:// chmai.loxinfo.co.th/helpage/Publication/Newage.htm#GREETNGS

Nkoyoyo, M. 1995. *Poverty and the elderly in Uganda: Cause and effect.* World Summit on Social Development, March, Copenhagen, Denmark. On-line: http://www.globalaging.org/resources/copenhagen/bishop.htm

Paul, J. 1995. *The worldwide pension crisis and "social development."* Presented at the World Summit on Social Development, Copenhagen, Denmark. On-line:

http://www.globalaging.org/resources/copenhagen/jpaul.htm

Paul, S., and J. Paul. 1995. The World Bank and the attack on pensions in
the global South. *International Journal of Health Services* 25 (4): 697–725.
On-line: http://www.globalaging.org/pension/world/pensions.htm

Population Division of the Department of Economic and Social Affairs at the
United Nations, Secretariat (UNPD-DESA). 1998. *World population projections to 2150*. February, United Nations, New York. On-line: http://www.
undp.org/popin/wdtrends/exesum.htm

Population Division of the Department for Economic and Social Information
and Policy Analysis of the United Nations Secretariat (UNPD-DESIPA).
1996. *Demographic impact of HIV/AIDS*. November, United Nations,
New York. On-line: http://www.undp.org/popin/wdtrends/demoimp.html

———. 1997. *World demographic trends: Report of the secretary general*. Presented
at the Thirteenth Session of the Commission on Population Development,
February, United Nations, New York.

Sadik, N. 1996. In spite of poverty: The older population builds towards the
future. Symposium conducted by the American Association of Retired Persons, the African American Institute, and the UNCHS (habitat), March,
New York.

United Nations Department of Public Information (UNDPI). 1996.
International year of older persons: The aging of the world's population
(DPI/1858/AGE). Online: http://www.un.org/ecosocdev/geninfo/aging/
aging-e.htm

United Nations Publications. 1996. United Nations Department for Economic
and Social Information and Policy Analysis, Population Division, International Migration Policy 1995. New York: United Nations. On-line:
http://www.undp.org/popin/wdtrends/migpol95/impieu.txt
http://www.undp.org/popin/wdtrends/migpol95/impina.txt
http://www.undp.org/popin/wdtrends/migpol95/impioc.txt
http://www.undp.org/popin/wdtrends/migpol95/impilac.txt
http://www.undp.org/popin/wdtrends/migpol95/impias.txt
http://www.undp.org/popin/wdtrends/migpol95/impiaf.txt

U.S. Bureau of the Census. 1995. *Statistical abstracts of the United States*. Washington, D.C.: GPO.

U.S. Bureau of the Census, International Population Reports. 1992. *An aging
world II*. P25, 92–93. Washington, D.C.: GPO.

U.S. Bureau of the Census, International Programs Center and International

Data Base. 1996. *Global aging into the 21st century* (wallchart). Washington, D.C.: Office of the Demography of Aging, Behavioral and Social Research Program, and National Institute on Aging.

CHAPTER TWO

Aging in America

This chapter presents the demographics of older persons in America, including the baby boomers and the old-old and the characteristics of racial and ethnic groups, specifically African Americans, Hispanic Americans, Asian Americans, and American Indians.

Population rates in some states and cities illustrate the migration patterns of older persons and areas with heavy concentrations of older persons. *Counter migration* refers to older persons who migrate to the Sunbelt from the Snowbelt, and those who return from the Sunbelt to be with family members. *Aging in place* refers to older persons who remain in communities where they lived most of their lives. Some questions explored in this chapter are:

- ❖ Will older persons continue to move to the Sunbelt areas of the United States as they have previously and, if so, which states are experiencing an aging growth?
- ❖ What is the social and economic impact of this unprecedented growth?
- ❖ What are the concerns of aging Americans?

Growth in the Population of Older Americans

At the beginning of the twenty-first century, 34.7 million people in the United States, 13% of the total population, were 65 years and older. Among these older persons, 20 million were ages 65–74 years, 11 million were 75–84 years, and 3.7 million were 85 years and older. America is experiencing tremendous growth in its older population. In 2030, the 65 and older population will be 20% of the total population of the United States (Dunker and Greenberg 1998). The growth in the population of those older than 65 years from 1900 to 2030 is illustrated in table 2.1.

In 1900, only 3.1 million Americans were 65 years or older and by 1920 this number had grown to 4.9 million. By 1960, there were 16.7 million Americans who were 65 years or older; by 2000 this number

Table 2.1 Growth of the Elderly Population (65 years and older)

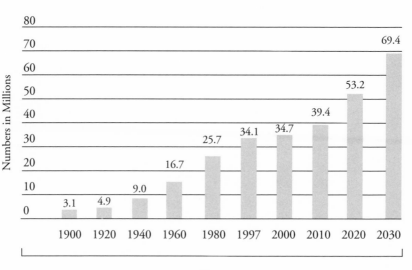

Year

Note: Increments in years are uneven

Source: Administration on Aging, 1998 (based on data from U.S. Bureau of the Census)

more than doubled to 34.7 million. Predictions for the year 2010 are that 39.4 million people will be 65 years of age or older; by 2030 this number will rise to 69.4 million (Dunker and Greenberg 1998). In 1996, while thirty nations had elderly populations of at least 2 million, the United States ranked third with 33.2 million. India was second with 36.3 million and China was first with 71.1 million (U.S. Bureau of the Census 1996a).

The Old-Old

The old-old are persons 85 years and older. This group is the fastest-growing group in America and worldwide. From 1960 to 1994 the number of those older than 85 years increased by 274%.

The United States Census Bureau projects an increase in the population age 100 years and older. In 1990, it was estimated that 37,306 Americans were age 100 years or older while in 2000 more than 72,000 people were centenarians. The centenarian population is expected to be 477,000 by 2030 (Hooyman and Kiyak 1996). Centenarian studies at the University of Georgia have identified specific factors that are common in persons 100 years and older in studies of physical health, functioning activity, cognitive performance, food patterns, dairy product intake, and nutritional habits. A more detailed explanation of the studies can be obtained from The University of Georgia Gerontology Center, Athens, Georgia (Holtsberg and Pugh 1994), but common characteristics of centenarians include a sense of optimism, a sense of humor, and a positive outlook. Studies of centenarians are ongoing in Denmark and in Finland. The twin studies of centenarians in those countries are searching for genetic links to longevity (Hooyman and Kiyak 1996).

The Division of Aging of Harvard Medical School is conducting a genetic study called the Centenarian Sibling Pair Study to determine whether or not centenarians and their family members share genes that may be related to diseases such as Alzheimer's disease, cancer, and heart disease (Koster and Prather 1999). The Harvard study is trying to determine if there is a centenarian personality. Margery Silver, lead author of this study, found that female centenarians were more likely to "be secure, hardy, and generally relaxed even under stressful conditions" (Miller 1999, 15). She stated, "What we noticed in working with these centenarians is that even those who had experienced a lot of stress in their lives were able to roll with the punches and were able to handle loss" (Miller 1999, 15).

The Baby Boomers

The number of older adults is expected to increase in the future as the baby boomers reach 65 years and older. The baby boomers are a cohort of individuals who were born between 1946 and 1964. The first of the baby boomers reached age 50 in 1996. The baby-boom generation will reach age 65 in the period from 2011 to 2030. This cohort of 75 million persons will substantially change aging as it is currently experienced because of their different life experiences and expectations. New technology and improved health status will impact the social and economic trends of this generation. By 2025, baby boomers will be between 61 and 79 years of age and ready for retirement (Campbell 1996). The retirement trends of the baby boomers suggest a cohort that will retire early and pursue varied leisure activities. The baby boomers are a group that matured in a period of economic growth in the United States and in other countries such as Australia and New Zealand. The developments in health care, communications technology, and education produced a cohort in better health and with better educations. Communications technology via the Internet has offered an unprecedented opportunity for baby boomers to learn from global sources. Communication with cohorts in Europe, Australia, Africa, Asia, and North and South America offers new opportunities for learning, personal development, and social planning. It is a simple task to research health events, health issues, and health research from global sources. Access to shopping sources may enhance the lifestyle of individuals with limited transportation or resources. Personal communications on the Internet for special-interest groups and family members can change relationships between family members who live in different areas or countries. The baby boomers will be a generation of technology users in their old age and they will change markets, create new businesses, influence politicians, and create new methods for the delivery of social services.

Racial and Ethnic Composition

Minority populations will represent 25% of the elderly population in 2030. In 1997, the minority population comprised 15% of the older population. Between 1997 and 2030, the white, non-Hispanic population ages 65 and older will increase by 91% compared to an expected increase of 328% for older minority persons.

Expected increases in older ethnic populations between 1997 and 2030 are:
 ❖ Hispanics – 570%
 ❖ Non-Hispanic blacks – 159%
 ❖ American Indians, Eskimos, and Aleuts – 294%
 ❖ Asian and Pacific Islanders – 643%

In 1996, the percentage of the total older adult population in America was 12.5%. The ethnic and racial groups were:
 ❖ Blacks – 8%
 ❖ Asian and Pacific Islanders – 2%
 ❖ American Indian or Native Alaskan – less than 1%
 ❖ Hispanics – 4.9%

These emerging elderly ethnic groups will bring new issues for an aging America (Dunker and Greenberg 1998).

African Americans

African Americans are the largest minority group (37 million) in the United States. Approximately 2.7 million, 8% of the total population, are older than 65 years (U.S. Bureau of the Census 1996a). About 53% of African Americans live in the South (Barrow 1996). The young outnumber the old due to the higher mid-life mortality rate of blacks (Hooyman and Kiyak 1996). Females outnumber males but the overall African American population 85 years and older will increase from 230,183 in 1990 to 1.4 million by 2050 (Dunker and Greenberg 1998).

African American elders are less likely to be married than any other ethnic group. The African American middle class now outnumbers the poor. Black elders have less income and poorer housing than their white counterparts. In 1992, 24.9% of older African Americans lived in poverty, triple that of white older persons. African Americans are less likely to have accumulated savings and to have assets such as real estate or pensions. Older African American persons retired from owning businesses or from employment as schoolteachers or government employees. Many African Americans retired from manual labor and service jobs. Older male African Americans have higher unemployment rates than do white older men. Older African Americans are more likely to be living in decaying urban areas and in substandard housing.

Life expectancy is lower for African Americans than for their white counterparts. African Americans tend to have more health problems. Life expectancy for the African American male is 64.6 years and for females it is 73.8 years. Between 1986 and 1991, life expectancy for African Americans dropped somewhat (Barrow 1996). One of the reasons for this drop is a high infant mortality rate for African Americans. African Americans often do not have adequate access to health care, which might reduce morbidity and mortality. The incidence of high blood pressure among African Americans is two and one-half times that of whites.

More than 40% of African American women older than 65 years live in poverty. High mortality rates of males and high divorce rates contribute to the poverty of African American women. African American older women provide help to other family members in caregiving and care of grandchildren and other extended family members. Religion is a major source of support in the lives of African Americans; the church has a long tradition of providing support and social services (Taylor 1993). African Americans tend to underutilize nursing homes and prefer care by family members. Select social and economic characteristics are reported in table 2.2.

Hispanic Americans

Hispanic Americans are the fastest-growing population group in the United States. Hispanic Americans include Mexicans, Puerto Ricans, Cubans, Central and South Americans, and the native Mexican Americans or Chicano population. The Hispanic population is a youthful group with a median age of 26.1 years. Only 4.9% of the Hispanic population, 1.9 million people, is older than 65 years. In 2010 this group is projected to be 2.9 million persons. If the trend continues, in 2030 the number of Hispanic elderly (7.6 million) will be larger than the black elderly population (6.8 million). This group also has a lower life expectancy than their white counterparts.

Higher percentages of Hispanic elderly, living below the poverty level, have poor health care and have achieved low occupational status, being primarily farm workers and laborers. Hispanics migrated to various locations in the United States and live in Los Angeles, New York, Chicago, Miami, Boston, Philadelphia, San Diego, San Antonio, Dallas, and Houston. Major linguistic barriers account for financial

Table 2.2 Social and Economic Characteristics of African Americans (1998)

Characteristic	Percentage
Age 65+	8.3
Homeowner	42.3
College, 4 years or more	11.9
Income of $50,000+	14.9
Unemployed	8.9

Source: U.S. Bureau of the Census, 1998

disadvantages of older Hispanics in regard to pensions and health-care access. Familism is common in Hispanic cultures and refers to strong family values. Adult children usually care for aged parents. Folk-healing beliefs and practices present a barrier in access to health care and may contribute to poor health care and higher rates of mortality and morbidity (Barrow 1996).

Asian Americans

Asian Americans are of various origins, including Korean, Chinese, Japanese, Filipino, East Indian, Thai, Vietnamese, Burmese, Indonesian, Laotian, Malayan, and Cambodian. The 1990 Census reports more than thirty subgroups. There are large concentrations of Asian Americans in California, Hawaii, New York, Illinois, and Washington. About 6% of the Asian American population is older than 65 years, or 0.5 million persons. The total Asian population in the United States, 7.5 million in 1990, increased rapidly due to the repeal of quotas in 1965. In contrast to other ethnic groups, Asian American men living alone constitute a large percentage of this ethnic group (Hooyman and Kiyak 1996).

Asian American older adults face language and cultural barriers in accessing health and social services. As a group, Asian Americans vary as to their cultural origins and the time of arrival in the United States. Recent waves of immigration have implications for family disorganization and economic development of the groups (Taylor 1998).

Japanese Americans immigrating to the United States in 1870 and 1924 were single men. Japanese Americans rapidly advanced economically and their children, born between 1910 and 1940, are now 65 and older and may well have achieved higher socioeconomic status. Chinese Americans were primarily single men who came in the early 1900s to work in the gold mines, farms, and railroads. The second generation of Chinese Americans is retiring with pensions and savings achieved from high occupational status. In recent years, the group of refugees from Cambodia, Vietnam, and Laos has included small numbers of older persons who are less educated. The low mean age of the Vietnamese American population and the Korean American population suggests that these groups will differ in socioeconomic status from current Chinese and Japanese populations. The median age for Japanese Americans is 36.3 years, suggesting that larger proportions of older persons may need support (Taylor 1998).

Greater numbers of workers per household and the practice of pooling resources for housing, schooling, and other needs accounts for the income advantage of Asian American families. While recent immigrants tend to be young adults of childbearing age, previous groups are aging in place. Changes and conflicts of traditional supports of the American-born generation are developing. Asian Americans are a cultural group that can be expected to have a major influence on American society.

American Indians/Native Americans

The 1990 Census reported 2 million American Indians of all ages in the total United States population of 248.7 million. Native Americans made up less than 1% of the total United States population. Older Indians comprised 8% of the 2 million American Indians of all ages. The total population of American Indians ages 60 and older was 166,000 in 1990 (Williams 1997). In 1992, this group had a median age of 26.5 years (Kart 1997). However, the number is projected to be more than 12.6% in 2050. The proportion of older persons in the American Indian population has grown faster than in other minority groups (Hooyman and Kiyak 1996). Between 1970 and 1980, their numbers increased by 6%.

Table 2.3 Asian American Groups in the United States

Pacific Islanders	Asian
Polynesian	Chinese
Hawaiian	Filipino
Samoan	Japanese
Tongan	Korean
Micronesian	Vietnamese
Guamanian	Laotian
	Thai
	Cambodian
	Pakistani
Source: Barrow, 1996	Indonesian

Native Americans have the lowest life expectancy of all minority groups. The average life expectancy for Native Americans is 65 years, or seven years less than the white population (Hooyman and Kiyak 1996). Native Americans are a diverse group, consisting of many different tribes with various customs and languages. In the United States, there are more than 300 recognized tribes (Barrow 1996). Native Americans remain a rural population. Fifty-three percent live in non-metropolitan areas, 22% live in central cities, and the remainder live in suburban areas. The census reports that elder Indians are nearly twice as likely to be rural dwellers compared to the total United States older population (48% versus 25%). The Native American population is concentrated in a few states. Nearly half, 45%, of older Indians live in just four states: Arizona, 9%; California, 13%; New Mexico, 6%; and Oklahoma, 17%.

Native American women outlive Native American men in every age group. More than 66% of older Native Americans live with family members. Literacy remains a problem for Native Americans. Unemployment, lack of education, and high rates of school dropouts create major difficulties for those who are growing old. Poverty and joblessness are lifetime problems. Chronic illnesses and disabilities are prevalent among this ethnic group. Native Americans are more likely to die of diabetes, alcoholism, pneumonia, suicide, and homicide. Accident rates are high. Reluctance to use health-care services is a major barrier to prevention of age-related diseases. Only 50% of older persons receive Social Security and Medicare benefits. Long-term care is usually provided by family members. The cost of long-term care for most groups will escalate and federal and state governments will be challenged to provide the services that older adults need to maintain a satisfactory quality of life.

States and Cities with Concentrations of Older Adults

It is expected that population will grow in the South, West, and the Northeast and decline in the Midwest. From 1995 to 2025, the South and the West will account for 82% of the 72 million people added to the United States population during this time. The South will grow due to increases in the birth rate, high domestic migration, and high international migration (Campbell 1996). The increase in the number of older persons is apparent, with Florida expecting an 8.3% increase, Arizona an 8.3% increase, North Carolina a 7.8% increase, South Carolina a 7.6% increase, and Nevada a 7.3% increase (U.S. Bureau of the Census 1996a).

Major graying areas are the South and West, which show the greatest gains in older adults migrating into those areas, while the Midwest and Northeast show the greatest losses in older adults due to the numbers leaving those areas. Florida, California, and New York have the largest elderly populations, with more than two million each. New Jersey, Pennsylvania, Illinois, Ohio, Michigan, and Texas each have more than one million older persons. Alaska has the smallest proportion of its population older than 65 years (4.1%), or 22,500 elderly residents (see table 2.7) (U.S. Bureau of the Census 1996a). From 1990 to 1995, the over-60 group grew 12% in Hawaii to 194,750 (U.S. Bureau of the Census 1996b).

Eight states (Nevada, Arizona, Colorado, Georgia, Alaska, Washington, Utah, and California) are expected to double their 65 and older population from 1993 to 2020. Nevada is the fastest-growing state in older adult population. Populations are aging because of in-migration, moving within the state, and because of out-migration of the young. A sustained low fertility rate is contributing to aging populations. In 1993, nine states had more than one million older persons (65 and older); however, the U. S. Census Bureau predicts that nineteen states will have more than one million older persons by the year 2020. The older population is less likely to change residence than other age groups. In 1994, only 6% of persons 65 and older moved, compared to 18% of those younger than 65 years of age.

Table 2.4 Regional Increases in the 65 and Older Population

Region	1995	2010	2025
U.S.	12.8%	13.2%	18.5%
Northeast	14.2%	13.7%	18.2%
Midwest	13.1%	13.6%	19.1%
West	11.3%	11.7%	16.1%
South	12.7%	13.8%	20.0%

Source: Campbell, 1996

Table 2.5 The 65 and Older Population by State, 1996

State	1996 Numbers (000's)	1996 Percent of Population Ages 65+	1990–1996 Percent Increase
U.S. Total	33,861	12.8	8.9
Alabama	557	13.0	7.2
Alaska	31	5.2	41.5
Arizona	586	13.2	23.1
Arkansas	362	14.4	3.9
California	3,516	11.0	13.0
Colorado	385	10.1	17.1
Conneticut	470	14.3	5.9
Delaware	93	12.8	15.2
District of Columbia	75	13.9	-2.1
Florida	2,657	18.5	11.2
Georgia	730	9.9	12.2
Hawaii	153	12.9	9.1
Idaho	135	11.4	11.7
Illinois	1,486	12.5	3.9
Indiana	735	12.6	5.9
Iowa	433	15.2	5.9
Kansas	352	13.7	2.9
Kentucky	489	12.6	5.2
Louisiana	497	12.6	6.4
Maine	173	13.9	6.5
Maryland	578	11.4	12.3
Massachusetts	859	14.1	5.4
Michigan	1,193	12.4	8.1
Minnesota	577	12.4	5.7
Mississippi	333	12.3	4.3
Missouri	742	13.8	3.7
Montana	116	13.2	9.2
Nebraska	229	13.8	2.7

Table 2.5 (continued)

State	1996 Numbers (000's)	1996 Percent of Population Ages 65+	1990–1996 Percent Increase
Nevada	183	11.4	44.9
New Hampshire	140	12.0	12.1
New Jersey	1,100	13.8	7.3
New Mexico	189	11.0	16.8
New York	2,434	13.4	4.0
North Carolina	917	12.5	14.6
North Dakota	93	14.5	2.7
Ohio	1,497	13.4	6.7
Oklahoma	445	13.5	5.3
Oregon	430	13.4	10.2
Pennsylvania	1,912	15.9	5.0
Rhode Island	156	15.8	4.3
South Carolina	447	12.1	8.3
South Dakota	105	14.4	3.3
Tennessee	667	12.5	8.3
Texas	1,951	10.2	14.2
Utah	175	8.8	17.3
Vermont	71	12.1	8.2
Virginia	747	11.2	13.0
Washington	641	11.6	11.9
West Virginia	278	15.2	3.7
Wisconsin	686	13.3	5.5
Wyoming	54	11.2	15.0

Based on data from the U.S. Bureau of the Census

Table 2.6 Eight States with the Fastest-Growing Elderly Population, 1993–2020 (number in thousands)

State	1993	2020	Percent Change
Nevada	155	333	115.6
Arizona	529	1,121	111.9
Colorado	357	743	108.0
Georgia	695	1,419	104.0
Washington	612	1,245	103.5
Alaska	26	54	103.3
Utah	165	334	102.4
California	3,303	6,622	100.5

Source: U.S. Bureau of the Census, 1996a

Table 2.7 States by Percentage of Population Ages 65 and Older, 1990

States	Percentage
Florida	18.3
Arkansas, Iowa, Pennsylvania, Rhode Island, South Dakota, West Virginia	14.7–15.4
Kansas, Missouri, Nebraska, North Dakota, Oregon	13.8–14.3
Arizona, Conneticut, Maine, Massachusetts, Montana, New Jersey, New York, Ohio, Oklahoma, Wisconsin	13.0–13.6
Alabama, Delaware, District of Columbia, Idaho, Kentucky, Illinois, Indiana, Minnesota, Mississippi, North Carolina, Tennessee	12.0–12.9
Louisiana, Michigan, Hawaii, New Hampshire, South Carolina, Vermont, Washington	11.1–11.9
California, Colorado, Georgia, Maryland, Nevada, New Mexico, Texas, Virginia, Wyoming	10.0–10.8
Utah	8.7
Alaska	4.1

Source: Kart, 1997

Table 2.8 U.S. Cities and Percent of Persons Older than 65 Years of Age

Cities	Percent of Population
Albany, N.Y.	14.6
Barnstable-Yarmouth, Mass.	22.8
Port Arthur, Tex.	13.2
Binghamton, N.Y.	14.7
Boston-Worcester-Lowell, Mass.	13.2
Buffalo-Niagara, N.Y.	15.7
Charleston, W. Va.	15.0
Chico-Paradise, Calif.	18.6
Cleveland-Akron, Ohio	14.3
Cumberland, Md.	18.9
Davenport-Moline, Ill.	16.6
Daytona Beach, Fla.	23.2
Decatur, Ill.	14.7
Duluth, Minn.	16.9
Eau Claire, Wis.	13.3
Elmira, N.Y.	15.6
Enid, Okla.	15.7
Fayetteville, Ark.	14.1
Florence, Ala.	14.8
Fort Myers, Fla.	24.8
Fort Pierce, Fla.	23.4
Gadsden, Ala.	16.3
Grand Junction, Colo.	14.7
Harrisburg, Pa.	14.1
Hartford, Conn.	14.1
Huntington-Ashland, W. Va.	14.5
Jamestown, N.Y.	16.3
Johnson City, Tenn.	14.9
Johnstown, Pa.	18.7
Lewiston-Auburn, Maine	14.2
Lynchburg, Va.	14.8

Table 2.8 (continued)

Cities	Percent of Population
Medford-Ashland, Ore.	15.7
Miami–Fort Lauderdale, Fla.	16.9
Myrtle Beach, S.C.	13.5
Naples, Fla.	22.4
Long Island, N.Y.	13.4
Ocala, Fla.	22.1
Parkersburg-Marietta, W. Va.	14.7
Pittsburgh, Pa.	17.7
Pittsfield, Mass.	17.7
Providence, R.I.	15.9
Pueblo, Colo.	15.4
Punta Gorda, Fla.	34.3
Redding, Calif.	15.0
Roanoke, Va.	16.1
San Luis Obispo–Atascadero, Calif.	15.1
Sarasota-Bradenton, Fla.	30.9
Scranton–Wilkes-Barre, Pa.	19.9
Sharon, Pa.	17.8
Sherman-Denison, Tex.	17.8
Sioux City, Iowa	14.0
South Bend, Ind.	14.2
Springfield, Ill.	14.0
Springfield, Mass.	14.4
Steubenville, Ohio	17.2
Tampa, St. Petersburg, Fla	21.9
Terre Haute, Ind.	15.9
Texarkana, Tex.	14.3
Tyler, Tex.	14.0
West Palm Beach–Boca Raton, Fla.	24.3
Williamsport, Pa.	15.8
Youngstown, Pa.	16.2

Source: http://www.census.Gov/Press-Release/metro09.prn
Data based on U.S. Bureau of the Census, 1997–98

In 1996, about 52% of persons 65 and older lived in nine states. California had more than 3 million; New York and Florida had about 2 million; and Texas, Pennsylvania, Ohio, Illinois, Michigan, and New Jersey had more than one million. In 1996, in more than ten states, more than 14% of the total population were persons older than 65 years. Florida has the largest proportion of older persons in the country (19%), and in 2025 it will remain the largest with 26% (Campbell 1996).

The U.S. Bureau of the Census reports several cities with populations older than 65 years that are greater than the national figure of 13% (see table 2.8). Older adults in rural areas are generally more disadvantaged because the rural older person tends to be isolated and have limited services. In spite of the myth that country living is synonymous with a better quality of life, the older person in metropolitan areas tends to be more active and in better health (U.S. Bureau of the Census 1998).

Migration Patterns

Most older people do not move. Persons ages 65 and older represented only 4% of all movers in the United States between 1992 and 1993. About 1.7 million older adults (non-institutionalized) moved to another house in the United States between 1992 and 1993. Only 1% moved to another state. Forty-nine percent of those who moved during 1992 and 1993 remained in the same metropolitan area, suggesting that most older persons stayed in the same region of the country where they had lived the year before.

In the Northeast, from 1992 to 1993 about 131,000 older persons moved from one county to another, 82% came from another county within the Northeast, and only 18% came from some other part of the country. About one-fourth of migrants in the Midwest (23%), the South (26%), and the West (30%) came from other regions. An analysis of the migrants indicates that older migrants tended to move to areas with a lower cost of living, less crime, and where family and friends reside.

The central cities of metropolitan areas lost older persons to non-metropolitan areas. Patterns of migration indicate that one pattern is amenity-motivated and the other is assistance-motivated. The old-old (ages 85 and over) were more likely to have moved than the young-old (65–74). The moves of the old-old may be health-related. There is also a rise in the migration patterns of females in very old age, which is associated with the prevalence of widowhood among this age group (Dunker and Greenberg 1998).

The volume of movement of older persons increased from 4.5 million between 1955 and 1960, to 5.8 million between 1975 and 1980, and 6.9 million between 1985 and 1990. While there was an increase in the number of interstate migrants, the number of intrastate migrants remained the same from 1985 to 1990. The economic implications of such migration are of concern to states in which out-migration has been the source of their economic losses, and states that received the older migrants are concerned about whether the gain in retirement income will offset the cost of health and social services for new elderly. During 1965–1970, 1975–1980, and 1985–1990, Florida was the state with the largest in-migration while New York was the state that had the largest out-migration (Dunker and Greenberg 1998).

Social and Economic Characteristics of Older Americans

Older Americans are not a homogenous group. There are differences in social characteristics and economic status. Aging differs for men and women, for ethnic groups, and for those who have a higher socioeconomic status.

Gender

In 1930, men and women were equal in number. In 1994, there were four elderly women to three elderly men worldwide. The world had 50 million more elderly women than men. By ages 80 and older, the world's women outnumber men two to one.

In 1994, 72% of those older than 85 in the United States were women. The general trend in survivorship of women is illustrated around the world. By 2050, the sex ratio of the old-old will be 60 to 100. There will be 4.7 million more women than men in this age group (Dunker and Greenberg 1998).

The combined factors of men generally being older than their spouses and the higher life expectancy of women contribute to the high proportion of women who live alone, are poor, and are institutionalized earlier than men. In addition, elderly women tend to be more of the poor in the country. Women are more than 70% of the older poor. Half of women older than 65 years are widows. The death of a spouse exposes a woman to economic risks. The opportunity for remarriage is limited since older women outnumber men. About 7% of women older than 60 are divorced. Eleven percent of those married for 20 years will divorce. Divorce negatively affects the socioeconomic status of women (Dunker and Greenberg 1998).

Poverty

The ten states with the highest poverty rates for older persons over the period 1993–1995 were:

* Mississippi (20%)
* Tennessee (20%)
* The District of Columbia (19%)
* Arkansas (19%)
* South Carolina (19%)
* Louisiana (18%)
* Alabama (17%)
* North Carolina (16%)
* Georgia (16%)
* South Dakota (15%)

In 1996, 10.8% of the 65 and older population were living in poverty, with an additional 7.8% considered "near poor." Women had a poverty rate of 13.6% and men a rate of 6.8%. More than 9% of 65 and older Caucasians, 25.3% of African Americans, and 24.4% of Hispanics were poor. In 1995, the median income for persons 65 and older was $16,684 for men and $9,626 for women. Major sources of income are:

* Social Security (92%)
* Property Assets (66%)
* Public and Private Pensions (32%)
* Earnings (16%)
* Public Assistance (5%)
  (Dunker and Greenberg 1998)

A poll conducted by Genesis ElderCare Corporation in 1997 found that Americans ages 80 or older reported being satisfied with their lives as often as those ages 65–69, but those with assets under $25,000 had lower levels of life satisfaction and a less positive view of aging (Genesis ElderCare).

Education

The population ages 65 and older is less likely to have completed high school than those persons ages 25 to 64 years. In 1993, elderly persons completing high school fell into the following categories:
- 60% of all elderly persons
- 67% of persons ages 65 to 69
- 52% of persons ages 75 and older
- 33% of older African American persons
- 38% of African American persons ages 65 to 74
- 23% of African American persons ages 75 and older
- 26% of older Hispanics

The educational attainment of the future elderly is expected to substantially increase. In 1993, 87% of persons ages 45 to 49 had at least a high school education; of persons ages 55 to 59, 77% had at least a high school education and 20% had a bachelor's degree. In 1990, 47% of older persons had not completed high school, while it is projected that in 2030 some 83% will have completed high school. The proportion of the elderly with a bachelor's degree will increase from 11% in 1990 to 24% in 2030 (Genesis ElderCare 1997).

Table 2.9 Educational Attainment of the Elderly by Sex, 1990

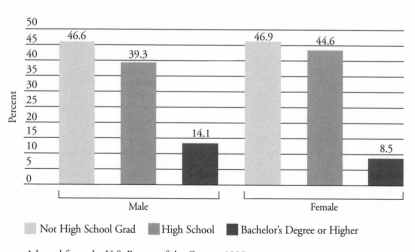

Not High School Grad   High School   Bachelor's Degree or Higher

Adapted from the U.S. Bureau of the Census, 1998

Table 2.10 Educational Attainment of the Elderly by Sex, 2030

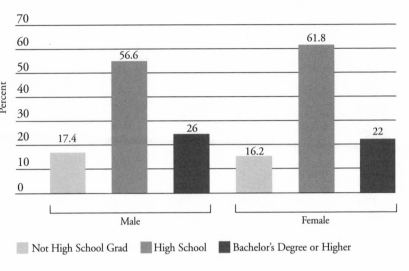

Adapted from the U.S. Bureau of the Census, 1998

Employment

The following facts indicate trends and changes in the employment participation of men and women in America.

1. Older workers have declined in the nation's work force.

2. In 1970, persons ages 55 years and older represented 19% of all workers while in 1993 they represented 13%.

3. There is a trend among men in their mid-fifties and early sixties to retire before they are of age to receive full retirement benefits.

4. The Bureau of Labor Statistics predicts that only 15% of men and 9% of women 65 years and older will be in the labor force in 2005.

5. While men retire from full-time employment in their fifties, they are increasingly returning to work part-time.

6. In 1967, 90% of men ages 55–59 were in the labor force while in 1993 78% were in the labor force.

7. In 1993, 38% of men ages 55 and older and 16% of men ages 65 and older were in the labor force.

8. Older men (75 and older) are increasingly less likely to be in the labor force.

9. Only 7% of men ages 75 and older are in the labor force.

10. African American men have lower rates of labor-force participation due to health and educational differences.

11. Only 5.3% of African American men older than 75 were employed in 1990.

12. Older women are more likely to work now than were older women in past generations.

13. In 1957, 38% of women in their thirties were in the labor force.

14. In 1993, 74% of women in their thirties were in the labor force.

15. While the level of participation of older men decreased, the level of participation of older women increased substantially.

16. For women ages 60 to 64, labor-force participation increased from 21% in 1950, to 36% in 1970, and 37% in 1993.

17. For women older than 65, labor-force participation rates remain low—from 10% in 1950, to 10% in 1967, and to 8% in 1993.

18. Older women participate in the labor force less than do older men. The rates dropped from 57% at ages 55–59, to 16% at ages 65–69, and to a low 3% for women ages 75 and older.

19. Older men are leaving the work force earlier than in previous years.

20. Larger proportions of older persons are in the work force part-time.

21. In 1993, about 54% of elderly workers were on part-time schedules.

22. More than 90% reported working voluntarily rather than for economic reasons.

23. The proportion of persons ages 55 and older working part-time in 1990 was 25%, compared to 19% in 1970.

24. Part-time employees are less likely to be covered by benefit programs such as health care and life insurance.

Marital Status

In 1995, older men were more likely to be married than older women; 76% of men and 43% of women were married in the United States. Half of all older women (65 and older) were widows. While the gender gap in longevity accounts for these differences, remarriage rates are also a factor. In 1990, only about 2 per 1,000 widowed women ages 65 and older remarried, while elderly men were more likely to remarry, about 14 in 1,000 (U.S. Bureau of the Census 1996a). Remarriage implies that elderly men will have a spouse when health fails and older women are not likely to have a spouse to provide care.

The number of divorced older persons increased (to 1.8 million) three times as fast as has the older population as a whole since 1990 (2.1 times for men and 4.2 times for women). In 1993, among all elderly men and women, about 5% were divorced and had not remarried. In 1990, only 30 of 1,000 divorced women remarried during the year. Divorced men are more likely to remarry than are divorced women. Little change in the proportion of married elderly females is expected well into the next century (Dunker and Greenberg 1998).

A common marital status for elderly women in the United States and in the world is widowhood. More than 35% of women ages 65 to 74 were widows in 1993. After age 75, the proportion of women who are widows increases substantially. About 59% of women ages 75 to 84 and about 79% of women ages 85 and older were widows in 1993. The likelihood for men is less, at 9% for men ages 65 to74, 19% for men ages 75 to 84, and 39% for men ages 85 and older. Black women are

Table 2.11 Marital Status of Persons 65 and Older, 1998

Data from the U.S. Bureau of the Census, 1998

more likely to become widows than white or Hispanic women in the same age group. Among Asian and Pacific Islanders, American Indians, Eskimos, and Aleuts, women are more likely to be widowed than are men. Among Asian and Pacific Islanders ages 75 and older, 68% of women were widowed while only 29% of men were widowed. Among American Indians, Eskimos, and Aleuts, 69% of women and 29% of men were widowed. Baby boom women are expected to experience widowhood later (Dunker and Greenberg 1998).

Concerns of Aging Americans

In a 1997 poll, older Americans were asked their concerns about aging. When asked if they see life as better or worse than twenty years ago, 35% see life as better, 38% see life as the same as twenty years ago, and 25% see it as worse. Asset level, marital status, and self-reported health status are more significant than age in determining if one sees life as better or worse than it was twenty years ago.

Interestingly, 50% of those Americans between ages 65–69 report that life is better now than at ages 45–49. Almost three-fourths of those 80 and older feel life is at least as good as it was twenty years earlier. Americans older than 65 identify the problems of the nation as one of their primary concerns. Next, they identify a group of personal concerns such as pains, mobility, vision, etc. Negative personal feelings such as loneliness and boredom are limited to 20% to 25% of all elders. Concern about money is highest among those 65–69 years. Older persons worry very little about death. They rated death as last among sixteen concerns of their lives. Data on why life is better today are reported in table 2.12.

Table 2.12 Why Life is Better Today: Reasons Reported by Elders (65 and older)

Characteristic	Percentage
Less stress/fewer worries	34%
More free time	28%
Financial security	21%
Able to be active	14%

Adapted from Genesis ElderCare, 1997

Table 2.13 Type of Help Received (65 and older) from Family Members

Emotional support	75%
Travel around	39%
Yard work	39%
Transportation	43%
Financial assistance	20%
Cleaning the house	30%
Shopping	40%
Preparing foods	26%

Adapted from Genesis ElderCare, 1997

Table 2.14 Concerns of Older Americans (65 and older)

Losing family and friends	63%
Not being able to walk as much	39%
Not being able to get around as well	35%
Note being able to do household chores as well	32%
Not having their children nearby	29%
Not traveling as much	27%
Not being able to play sports as well	24%
Not being as sexually active	22%
Losing their looks	21%
Not having a job	18%
Not having access to shopping	18%
Not being independent	16%

Adapted from Genesis ElderCare, 1997

Older adults of all ages report positive feelings about themselves. Negative self-feelings are expressed regarding activities that require mobility. At least 93% state that they look forward to each new day; 91% enjoy meeting new people, 77% indicate they are religious, and more than 60% report that they feel attractive.

Dependency is the primary negative feeling older adults have about themselves. The number one concern is, "I worry about being a burden on others." Issues of concern about functionality and mobility increase with age, especially after 80 years.

Fear of being mugged or robbed is not associated with age or community level. Those persons who live in rural areas are as concerned as older persons who live in urban areas.

Sixty-one percent of older Americans receive some type of help from their families. Family members are called upon to provide assistance. The level of support increases significantly for older persons whose assets are less than $25,000. More than two-thirds of older adults 65 years and older report good or excellent health status. Low self-reported health status is related to low life satisfaction. Low health status is also related to increased worry about functionality. The number of older persons who say their health is good or excellent does not differ significantly with age, sex, or living status but does vary by income. For example, 67% of men and 65% of women report good/excellent health. Sixty-seven percent of persons 65–69, 65% of persons 70–74, 68% aged 75–79 years, and 64% of persons 80 or older report good/excellent health. Sixty-nine percent who are married and 63% of those persons not married report good/excellent health.

Additionally, 67% of persons living with someone and 65% of persons living alone report good/excellent health. However, 84% of older persons with assets of more than $100,000, 70% of those persons with assets of $25,000–$99,000, and only 57% with assets of less than $25,000 report good/excellent health. Older persons worry more about their physical health than mental health (58% versus 36%) (Genesis ElderCare 1997).

Another study released by the National Council on Aging found that nearly half of older Americans say, "These are the best years of my life" (2000).

Summary

Americans will age in unprecedented numbers. The total elderly population will more than double. The Sunbelt states will continue to grow in population, with Nevada experiencing the greatest growth. Florida will have the largest percentage of older persons in the country. Migration of older persons to states offering amenities and a lower cost of living will increase. The major graying areas will be the South and West. Moving from Sunbelt to Frostbelt suggests another move after retirement (i.e., counter migration). Compared with those who move to the Sunbelt, those who move back to the Frostbelt are generally disabled or widowed. In the future, women are more likely to have pensions in their own names and more stable retirement income.

The trend toward early retirement for men seems likely to continue. More early retirees are working part-time and are referred to as "working retirees." Changes in pension plans will affect early retirement decisions. A decline in the proportion of widowed women is expected as men improve their chances of survival beyond age 65. Notable increases are expected in the proportion of divorced persons. Divorced baby boomers are less likely to remarry. Financial security in the earlier years seems to be related to health status and to future concerns in the later years. Americans are expected to be better educated, financially stable, and living healthier, more active life styles.

References

Barrow, G. 1996. *Aging, the individual, and society.* 6th ed. Los Angeles: West Publishing.

Campbell, P. 1996. *Population projections for states by age, sex, race, and Hispanic origins: 1995 to 2025.* U.S. Bureau of the Census, Population Division, PPL-47. On-line: http://www.census.gov/population/www/projections/pp147.html.

Dunker, A., and S. Greenberg. 1998. *A profile of older Americans: 1998.* Washington, D.C.: Program Resources Department, American Association of Retired Persons (AARP), and the Administration on Aging (AoA), U.S. Department of Health and Human Services. On-line: http://www.aoa.dhhs.gov/stats/profile/.

Genesis ElderCare. 1997. *A look at aging in America: The Genesis ElderCare poll.* Kennett Square, Pa.: Genesis ElderCare

Holtsberg, Philip A., and Katherine Pugh. 1994. *Georgia's centenarian: The quintessential positive model of aging?* Athens: Univ. of Georgia Press.

Hooyman, N., and H. A. Kiyak. 1996. *Social gerontology: A multidisciplinary perspective.* 4th ed. Boston: Allyn and Bacon.

Kart, Cary S. 1997. *The realities of aging: An introduction to gerontology.* 6th ed. Boston: Allyn and Bacon.

Koster, J., and J. Prather, eds. 1999. Global Aging e-Report. Electronic supplement of AARP *Global Aging Report.* On-line: http://www.aarp.org/intl/

Miller, Claudia. 1999. Personality: A clue to longevity? *Aging Today* 20 (1) (Jan./Feb.): 15.

National Council on Aging. 2000. Online: http://ncoa.org.news/mra_2000fact shet.html

Taylor, Robert J. 1993. Religion and religious observances. In *Aging in black America,* edited by J. S. Jackson, L. M. Chatters, and R. J. Taylor. Newberry Park, Calif.: SAGE Publications.

Taylor, Ronald L. 1998. Minority families and social change. In *Minority families in the United States,* edited by Ronald L. Taylor. Upper Saddle River, N.J.: Prentice Hall.

U.S. Bureau of the Census. 1996a. *Current Population Reports, Special Studies. P23–190, 65+ in the United States.* Washington, D.C.: GPO.

U.S. Bureau of the Census. 1996b. *U.S. Census Bureau: The official statistics.* On-line: http://www.census.gov/search97cgi/www.hawaii.gov/health/coa/kupuna.htm).

U.S. Bureau of the Census. 1997–98. *State and Metropolitan Area Data Book 1997–98.* On-line: http://www.census.gov/Press-Release/metro09.prn

U.S. Bureau of the Census. 1998. *Statistical abstracts of the United States.* Washington, D.C.: GPO.

Williams, B. S. 1997. *Native American elder population, 1990* (Based on Bureau of the Census Count). Washington, D.C.: Office for American Indian, Alaskan Native, and Native Hawaiian Programs, and U.S. Administration on Aging (AoA), and Department of Health and Human Services. On-line: http://www.aoa.dhhs.gov/ain/naepop90.html.

CHAPTER THREE

Life Expectancy

Increases in life expectancy will be remembered as a phenomenon of the twentieth century that changed the sociopolitical face of the world. *Life expectancy* is defined as the number of years, on average, that one can expect to live. *Life span* refers to the maximum limit of human life. Life expectancy has increased in North America, Europe, Asia, Australia, South America, and Africa. Increases in life expectancy will impact socioeconomic planning in developed and developing countries. Which countries have the highest average life expectancy and which countries have the lowest life expectancy? What biopsychosocial theories explain this phenomenon? What is active life expectancy?

Contributing factors to the unprecedented increase in global life expectancy are advances in medical technology, changes in health-care systems, and changes in lifestyle behaviors. New data emerge virtually every month regarding reasons for the increase in life expectancy globally. Scientists study animals and humans in laboratories worldwide to solve the puzzle of longevity. In America, the Baltimore Longitudinal Study began an investigation of healthy older persons in 1958, and in other countries the search for the key to the fountain of youth involves major research efforts.

Life Expectancy Worldwide

Global average life expectancy at birth in 1997 was 64.3 years (62.2 years for men and 66.5 years for women). On average, an individual born in a developed country can expect to outlive someone born in the developing world by more than eleven years. Improvements in life expectancy were more rapid in the first half of the century because of improvements in public health services. Disease eradication greatly reduced death rates, especially among infants and children. All nations showed an improvement in life expectancy rates. East Asia had the most impressive gains, with life expectancy increasing from the 1950 rate of less than 45 years to 71 years in 1990.

As female life expectancy continued to rise, male life expectancy leveled off. From the 1950s to the 1970s there was little change in male life expectancy in Australia, the Netherlands, Norway, and the United States. However, male life expectancy has increased again. Currently, women outlive men by five to nine years. Male mortality significantly surpasses female mortality at later stages of life. A dramatic increase in life expectancy worldwide occurred in the twentieth century and is expected to continue. Spain has more than doubled its average life expectancy from 35 years for women in 1900 to 81.8 years in 1990 (Bosch 1998).

Table 3.1 shows changes in average life expectancy at birth between 1960 and 1992. In 1960, Australia had a life expectancy of 72 years. In 1992, Australia's life expectancy increased to 78 years. Most countries had significant increases in life expectancy, with the exception of Mongolia and Russia, where life expectancy decreased. Life expectancy in Russia decreased from 1989 when it was 62 years to 58 years in 1999. Significant drops are noted in Armenia, Belarus, Bulgaria, Latvia, Lithuania, and Romania. The most immediate cause of the rising mortality is related to the rise in self-destructive behavior such as alcoholism and drug abuse. In addition, suicide rates rose sharply in Russia (60%) and in Lithuania (80%) (Ciment 1999).

Table 3.1 Average Life Expectancy at Birth: Changes in Selected Countries, 1960–1992

Country	Year	
	1960	**1992**
Australia	72.0	78.0
Canada	71.0	77.2
Singapore	64.5	74.2
Poland	67.1	71.5
Israel	68.6	76.2
Chile	57.1	71.9
Mongolia	67.9	63.0
Zimbabwe	56.7	56.2
India	45.3	59.7
Sierra Leone	44.0	60.9
Egypt	46.2	64.0

Adapted from UNDIESA, 1991

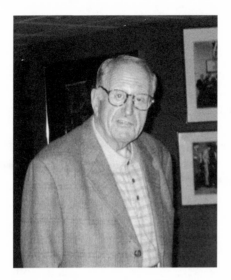

The age of 80 years is a time of distinction.

On average, one million people become 60 years old each month around the globe. Life expectancy in North America is 76.2 years; in Europe it is 72.7 years; in Oceania it is 72.9 years; in Africa it is 51.8 years; in Asia it is 64.5 years; in Latin America it is 68.5 years; and in the United States it is 76 years (UNPD-DESIPA 1997).

The U.S. Bureau of the Census reports that the projected life expectancy of individuals at birth in the year 2000 will be highest in North America, with Canada having the longest life expectancy of 79.1 years. France has the highest life expectancy in Europe at 79.2 years. Hong Kong's life expectancy is 80 years and Japan's life expectancy is 80.6 years. South America's life expectancy is highest in Paraguay at 74.9 years. Africa's longest life expectancy rate at birth is in Algeria at 69.6 years. Australia's life expectancy is 78.7 years (see table 3.2) (Kart 1997).

In New Zealand, life expectancy increased as a result of improved infant survival, better housing and public-health facilities, improved standards of living, improved nutrition, and improved medical care. The changes in life expectancy in New Zealand were notable. In 1950, women could expect to live to 71.3 years and men to 67.2 years. In 1987, women could expect to live to 77.1 years and men to 71.1 years (Koopman-Boyden 1993).

Table 3.2 Projected Life Expectancy at Birth for Selected Countries, 1994 and 2000

Country	1994	2000
North America	**76.2**	
Canada	78.1	79.1
Mexico	72.9	75.0
United States	75.9	76.4
Europe	**72.7**	
Denmark	75.8	77.4
Finland	75.9	77.4
France	78.2	79.2
Italy	77.6	78.7
Netherlands	77.8	78.8
Poland	72.7	75.0
Romania	71.7	74.4
Russia	68.9	70.5
United Kingdom	76.8	78.1
Asia		
China	67.9	70.2
Hong Kong	80.1	80.6
India	58.6	61.4
Japan	79.3	80.0
South America		
Brazil	62.3	60.9
Colombia	72.1	74.2
Paraguay	73.3	74.9
Peru	65.6	68.1
Africa		
Algeria	67.7	69.6
Ethiopia	52.7	55.4
Nigeria	55.3	59.1
South Africa	65.1	67.0
Australia	77.6	78.7
Middle East		
Israel	78.0	78.9
Saudi Arabia	67.9	71.1

Source: Kart, 1997

Table 3.3 Regional Life Expectancy: Africa (in years)

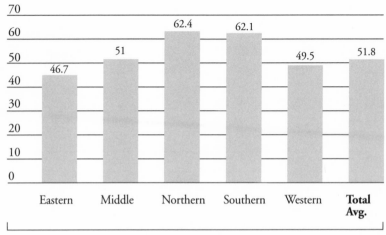

Source: UNPD-DESIPA, 1997

Table 3.4 Regional Life Expectancy: Asia (in years)

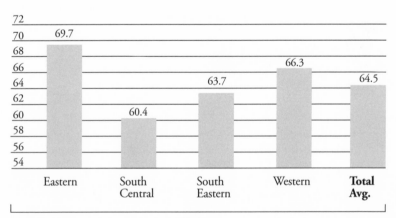

Source: UNPD-DESIPA, 1997

Table 3.5 Regional Life Expectancy: Latin America/Caribbean (in years)

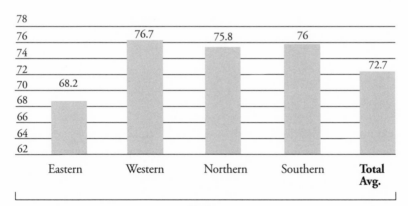

	Caribbean	Central America	South America	Total Avg.
	68.5	70.5	67.8	68.5

Region

Source: UNPD-DESIPA, 1997

Table 3.6 Regional Life Expectancy: Europe (in years)

	Eastern	Western	Northern	Southern	Total Avg.
	68.2	76.7	75.8	76	72.7

Region

Source: UNPD-DESIPA, 1997

Life expectancy remains lower in developing countries such as South Korea. In South Korea, life expectancy in 1990 was 68.2 years for males and 75 years for females. The growth rate of the Korean population declined from 2.9% in 1960 to 0.98% in 1990. This sharp decrease in population growth brought about the rapid increase of population aging (Rhee 1995).

Life Expectancy for the Old-Old

In Sweden, France, England, the United States, and Japan, life expectancy dramatically increased for people 80 years and older.

 ❖ American women who were 80 years of age could expect to live an average of 9.1 years; American men, an average of 7 or more years.
 ❖ Japanese women could expect to live an average of 8.5 years; Japanese men could expect to live 6.9 years.
 ❖ Swedish women, 8.3 years; Swedish men, 6.5 years.
 ❖ French women, 8.6 years; French men, 6.7 years.
 ❖ English women, 8.1 years; English men, 6.9 years.

Some explanations offered for Americans are:

 ❖ American older adults may be more demanding of high-quality health services.
 ❖ American older persons may receive more effective health care than do older persons in other countries.
 ❖ Higher mortality rates among younger people in the United States may leave a group of healthy survivors at advanced ages. (Beyond 80 1996, 1)

Countries with Highest and Lowest Life Expectancy

The countries with the lowest average life expectancy are Rwanda (22.6 years), Sierra Leone (34.4 years), and Uganda (41years). Japan and Hong Kong are the countries with the highest overall average life expectancy with an average of 80 years. France's average life expectancy is 79.2 years, Canada's is 79.1 years, and Iceland's is 78.9 years (UNPD-DESIPA 1997).

Differences in life expectancy are the result of high infant mortality rates, AIDS, disease, and war. Life expectancy in Taiwan increased to 72.4 years due to improvements in the environment and medical care

(Chang 1986). Globally, since the 1900s improvements in average life expectancy were very rapid during the first half of the century. Due to an almost universal decline in fertility and an increase in life expectancy, the growth of the older population is a worldwide phenomenon.

Africa remains low in life expectancy worldwide. Average life expectancy in Africa's regions range from a low of 46.7 years to a high of 62.1 years. In Asia, life expectancy ranges are from a low of 60.4 years to a high of 69.7 years. Average life expectancy is highest in Central America at 70.5 years, followed by the Caribbean at 68.5 years and South America at 67.8 years. Average life expectancy is higher in Europe than in most other regions, with the total average for all of Europe being 72.7 years. Western Europe has the longest life expectancy of 76.7 years, followed closely by Southern Europe with an average of 76 years, and Eastern Europe with 68.2 years (Global Aging Report 1997).

Life Expectancy in the United States

In 1997, the average life expectancy was 79.5 years for women and 72.5 years for men in the United States (U.S. Bureau of the Census 1996).

Table 3.7 Life Expectancy in the United States from 1900 to 1991

Year	Age (In Years)
1900	47.3
1920	56.6
1940	63.8
1950	68.2
1960	69.7
1970	70.8
1980	73.7
1991	75.5

Source: U.S. Bureau of the Census, 1996

In 1900, average life expectancy in the United States was 47.3 years; in 1920 it was 56.6 years; in 1940 it was 63.8 years, and it increased steadily until 1991 when it was 75.5 years. In 2050, men in the United States can expect to live to be 86 years of age and women can expect to live to 92 years of age (U.S. Bureau of the Census 1996). Overall, American women live the longest in Minnesota (83.5 years) and men live the longest in Utah (77.5 years). The worst counties for life expectancy were in South Dakota, where life expectancy for men was 61 years and for women 70 years. The ten least-healthy areas were in the South (Black men 1997).

Gender Differences in Life Expectancy

Women outlive men in all countries. Women's greater longevity and patterns of marrying older men create substantially higher proportions of women who live alone and who are poor when widowed. Older women are more likely than men to live in residential-care facilities. Women are more likely than men to need assistance in one or more functions of daily living such as toileting, bathing, mobility, eating, or dressing. Women are more likely to have chronic illnesses (U.S. Bureau of the Census, International Population Reports 1992).

In 1993, life expectancy was highest in the world for older persons in Japan. A Japanese man could expect to live 16.7 years beyond his sixty-fifth birthday; a Japanese woman could expect to live 21.3 years beyond her sixty-fifth birthday. France followed closely, and Hong Kong followed with an added 17.1 years for men and 20.8 years for women beyond the sixty-fifth birthday. In Sweden, Italy, and the United States, men can expect to live an additional 15.5 years and women 19.3 years beyond their sixty-fifth birthday.

In the Russian Federation, men can expect to live 10.9 years and women 15 years beyond their sixty-fifth birthday. In Australia, life expectancy beyond the sixty-fifth birthday is 13 years for women and 11 years for men (Australian Bureau of Statistics 1997).

In the 1950s, life expectancy rates began to change for men and women. Female life expectancy began to rise while male life expectancy began to level off from 1950 to the 1970s in the United States, Australia, and the Netherlands. All nations have shown improvement rates in life expectancy (except Russia), while the most impressive gains have been in East Asia (U.S. Bureau of the Census, International Population Reports 1992).

Although male life expectancy at birth increased in countries such as the United States and Australia, female life expectancy at birth in low-mortality societies such as Japan and Switzerland continues to outpace that of males. The gender gap in developing countries is three to six years.

Table 3.8 Years Expected to Live after Age 65 in Selected Countries (by sex)

Country	Males	Females
Japan	16.7	21.3
France	16.2	21.3
Hong Kong	17.1	20.8
Switzerland	15.9	20.4
Canada	15.8	19.9
Australia	15.8	19.7
Spain	15.2	19.7
Sweden	15.6	19.3
Italy	15.5	19.3
United States	15.5	19.3
Norway	14.8	18.8
Netherlands	14.4	18.8
Greece	16.0	18.7
New Zealand	15.0	18.6
Germany	14.5	18.3
Singapore	15.3	18.0
United Kingdom	14.2	18.0
Israel	15.8	17.7
Chile	14.7	17.6
Ireland	13.6	17.3
Poland	12.5	16.2
Russian Federation	10.9	15.0

Source: Australian Bureau of Statistics, 1967–94

Table 3.9 Life Expectancy at Birth for Males and Females in 1900, 1950, 1990

Country	1900		1950		1990	
	Male	*Female*	*Male*	*Female*	*Male*	*Female*
United States	48.3	51.1	66.0	71.7	72.1	79.0
Austria	37.8	39.9	62.0	67.0	73.5	80.4
Belgium	45.4	48.9	62.1	67.4	73.4	80.4
Denmark	51.6	54.8	68.9	71.5	72.6	78.4
England	46.4	50.1	66.2	71.1	73.3	79.2
France	45.3	48.7	63.7	69.4	73.4	81.9
Germany	43.8	46.6	64.6	68.5	74.5	80.6
Italy	42.9	43.2	63.7	67.2	74.5	81.4
Norway	52.3	55.8	70.3	73.8	73.4	80.8
Sweden	52.8	55.3	69.9	72.6	72.6	80.7
Czechoslovakia	38.9	41.7	60.9	65.5	65.5	76.5
Greece	38.1	39.7	63.4	66.7	66.7	80.2
Hungary	36.6	38.2	59.3	63.4	63.4	75.4
Poland	n/a	n/a	57.2	63.8	62.8	76.7
Spain	33.9	35.7	59.8	64.3	64.3	81.6
Australia	53.2	56.8	56.8	71.8	71.8	79.8
Canada	n/a	n/a	n/a	70.9	70.9	80.7
Japan	42.8	44.3	59.6	63.1	63.1	82.1
New Zealand	n/a	n/a	67.2	71.3	71.3	78.4

Source: UNDEISA, 1991

This trend is true in countries such as Austria, Italy, Sweden, Spain, Poland, and Japan. In 1950, the gap widened in Australia with men having an average life expectancy of 56.8 years and women 71.8 years. The gap was still evident in other countries in 1990. Japanese men had a life expectancy of 63.1 years, while women had an expectancy of 82.1 years. In Greece men had an average life expectancy of 66.7 years and women, 80.2 years (U.S. Bureau of the Census, International Population Reports 1992).

Average life expectancy for women is more than 80 years in at least fifteen countries. There are some indications that the gender gap in life expectancy is lessening. Research indicates that the gap remains in developing countries primarily due to alcohol and tobacco consumption and vehicular and industrial accidents. While the proportion of older women continues to grow steadily, women are more likely to be poorer, have more chronic long-term illnesses, need care, and become victims of elder abuse (U.S. Bureau of the Census, International Population Reports 1992).

Ethnic Differences in Life Expectancy

Being a member of a minority group is often associated with numerous risk factors in life, including poverty, poor health care, and psychological and physical health problems, all as a consequence of low income and stress. These disadvantages contribute to lower life expectancy rates in minority elders. In the United States, people of color—Native Americans, African Americans, Asian Americans, and Hispanics, who have physical and cultural characteristics that are different than Caucasians—are minority groups (Mui, Choi, and Monk 1998).

Overall African American elderly are more likely to suffer more illnesses and die earlier. They are more likely to have heart disease, high blood pressure, strokes, and diabetes. Coke and Twaite (1995) report that 51% of all African Americans who are 65 and older are limited in a major life activity by a chronic health condition. In 1993, African American males had an average life expectancy of 66 years; the average life expectancy of African American females was 74.7 years compared to that of white females at 79.5 years and for white males at 73.1 years.

A study in Washington, D.C., found that African American men in that city have a life expectancy of only 57.9 years, second only to male American Indians living in the worst South Dakota counties, who have a life expectancy of 56.5 years. Male Asian Americans in affluent communities in New York and Massachusetts live to be 89.5 years and Asian American women live to the mid-nineties. The life expectancy for older African American persons was reported to be 69.7 years in 1995 and projected to be 75.3 years in 2050 (Black men 1997).

For Hispanics the most common health problems are high blood pressure, arthritis, circulatory diseases, diabetes, cataracts, and heart disease. They are less likely than whites to die from the three major killers—heart disease, cancer, and stroke—and more likely to die from diabetes and liver disease. Mexican Americans have a lower infant mortality rate. Hispanic men are nearly twice as likely as white men to die from AIDS; Hispanic women are nearly five times as likely to die from the disease as white women. In 1995, life expectancy for Hispanics was 78.9 years. It is projected to be 87 years in 2050 (Zaldivar 1998).

In 1955, the general health of American Indian people was well behind the rest of the United States population and mortality rates were substantially higher. The life expectancy of American Indians and Alaskan Natives increased over the decades due to preventative health programs and changes in lifestyle behaviors. Life expectancy increased 20 years from 1940 to 1980. The death rate for Indian infants dropped 82%. In 1995 population projections, the life expectancy of American Indians, which includes American Indians, Eskimos, and Aleuts, was reported to be 76.2 years and projected to be 82.5 years in 2050 (Rhoades, D'Angelo, and Hurlburt 1987).

Another indigenous group that experiences the results of minority status are in Australia: the Australian Aborigines. For the Aborigines, life expectancy is considerably lower (66 years) than the majority population of white Australians (Australian Bureau of Statistics 1994). In New Zealand, the minority population of Maori also has lower rates of life expectancy than the majority white population. While Maori life expectancy has improved considerably in the twentieth century, it is still below the Pakeha (majority population): 7 years less for men and 8.5 years less for women. The number of Maori older than 65 years is expected to grow from the current population of 3.3% to 6.6% in 2011 (Koopman-Boyden 1993). Overall, minority groups in most countries experience lower rates of life expectancy.

Active Life Expectancy

An international network called REVES (the French acronym for the International Research Network for Interpretation of Observed Values of Health Life Expectancy) was formed to promote analysis of healthy life expectancy, or what is also known as active life expectancy. This network brings together researchers who measure changes in health status among nations. They produce a statistical yearbook that includes

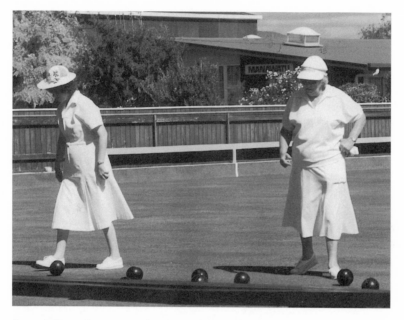

Lawn ball is a favorite social and physical activity for older women in New Zealand.

existing estimates of healthy life expectancy in various countries (REVES 1991).

Gerontologists make a distinction between *active life expectancy,* or *disability-free life expectancy,* and *life expectancy. Active life expectancy* is operationally defined by Kart (1997, 105) as "the period of life free of limitations in activities of daily living." How many years of active life can be expected?

It is difficult to compare healthy life expectancy among nations because computational methods differ and the concepts and definitions vary (Chamie 1997). Health status is measured in many ways, and there is little standardization of survey methods, leading to difficulty in comparing data. However, the REVES report states that, worldwide, time spent in good health after age 65 ranges from 45% to 80% for men and from 37% to 76% for women (REVES 1991). Women can expect to spend more years in a disabled state than men. The data also suggest that developing countries show a wide variation in the proportion of years after age 65 spent in good health. For men the range is from 60% to 88% and for women, the range of healthy remaining life is 50% to 87%.

A four-country study found that in Japan, the United States, and Great Britain, mortality decreased and morbidity increased, but in Hungary the opposite occurred (Riley 1990). Riley found that the risk of long-term illness has decreased due to earlier and better detection of sickness, declining mortality, and rising real income. In Australia, more than 80% of women survive to age 70, but only about half do so without some disability. Thus, the relationship between morbidity and mortality remains unclear. Gains in life expectancy have not led to improved overall health in many countries.

In a study in the Netherlands (Nusselder et al. 1996), researchers focused on the impact of eliminating lung disease, heart disease, cancer, diabetes, arthritis, and neurological diseases and found that, after eliminating lung disease or diabetes, there was an increase in disability-free life expectancy for women. Eliminating cancer, heart disease, and diabetes increased life expectancy for men but meant an increase in the proportion of life spent in disability.

Contrasting Perspectives on Extending Life

The effects on societies of extending life are yet uncertain. Will it be possible to support the increasing numbers of old people if they continue to age in the same manner of frailty and dependency? Can the world afford a dependent, sick, older population? Fries (1984) predicts a compression of morbidity whereby older persons will experience long, healthy, and active lives with short periods of morbidity before death. This perspective implies that future older people will have fewer debilitating illnesses and will experience only a few years of major illness in very old age, and death will occur due to the natural wearing out of all organ systems at around age 100.

Verbugge (1990) offers a contrasting perspective. She argues that with increasing numbers of older people there would be increases in the number of individuals with physical and mental health problems. Morbidity rates increased based on the National Health Interview Survey, which tracked morbidity rates from 1958 to 1985; older persons were living longer but with more disability and longer periods of restricted activity. There is some evidence that death from infectious disease has been replaced by death from degenerative diseases.

Summary

Increase of life expectancy will have a profound impact on all aspects of society. The increase in life expectancy, globally, is the result of decreases in infant mortality, decreases in adult mortality from infectious diseases such as pneumonia, and advances in medical technology. The challenge for most countries is how to improve the quality of life of the increased numbers of older persons. Life expectancy changed from 45 years in 1945, to 65 years in 1997, and we predict it will be 76 years in 2045 (Chamie 1997).

Average life expectancy will increase to about 90 years in most developed countries and will have a profound effect on health and social services and economic resources. The use of hospital services, residential-care services, hospice, and home-care services increases with age. Persons older than 65 years are major consumers of health-care services. This trend is expected to continue if older persons age into the future with the same amount of physical disabilities as the current older population; the demand on social services for respite care, counseling, psychiatric services, housing, financial assistance, and protection from elder abuse will be unprecedented in our history. The cost of home-care services is a major concern for most governments. We have increased the average life expectancy worldwide. We are now on the road to improving the quality of those added years.

Longevity and quality of life are the goals. The New England Centenarian Study, from Harvard Medical School, released a "life expectancy calculator" that is designed for individuals to estimate their longevity potential. Thomas Perls, M.D., M.P.H., argues that the average person is born with a set of genes that would allow him or her to live to be about 85 years or older, but preventive steps can add as much as ten years to that individual's life. The calculator has twenty-three items, which are answered with a yes or no. Some questions inquire about family history and environmental factors such as exposure to air pollution or levels of radon in the home; others refer to diet, exercise, stress, and personal hygiene. This questionnaire can be found on the Internet at http://www.livingto100.com (Perls 1999).

References

Australian Bureau of Statistics, Deaths in Australia for various years. 1967–94. Cat No. 3302.0. Canberra: Australian Government Publishing Service (AGPS).

Beyond 80. 1996. *People's Medical Society Newsletter* 15 (1) (Feb.): 6–7. Electronic Reference: University of South Carolina Infotrac Database, Health Reference center—Academic (Article A18137592).

Black men in D.C. have shorter life expectancy. 1997. *Jet* 93 (5) (Dec.): 18–19. Electronic Reference: University of South Carolina Infotrac Database, Health Reference Center—Academic (Article A20112979).

Bosch, Xavier. 1998. Spanish live long and healthy lives. *Lancet* (Nov.). Electronic reference: University of South Carolina Infotrac, Health Reference Center—Academic (Article A53247070).

Chamie, J. 1997. Statements to the Commission on Population and Development (thirtieth session). Speech presented to the meeting of the United Nations Commission on Population and Development, February, United Nations, New York.

Chang, J. L. 1986. Reflections from the field: Community services for the aged in Taipei. *Social Development Issues* 10 (2): 84–88.

Ciment, J. 1999. Life expectancy of Russian men falls to 58. *British Medical Journal* 319: 468.

Coke, M. M., and J. A. Twaite. 1995. *The black elderly: Satisfaction and quality of later life.* Binghamton, N.Y.: Haworth Press.

Consumer Reports on Health. 1995. *How long will you live? Take this test to see how many more years you can expect.* Electronic reference: University of South Carolina Infotrac Database, Health Reference Center—Academic (Article A17928506).

Fries, J. F. 1984. The compression of morbidity: Miscellaneous comments about a theme. *Gerontologist* 24: 354–59.

International Research Network for Interpretation of Observed Values of Healthy Life Expectancy (REVES). 1991. *Statistical World Yearbook.* Supplement to Bibliography Series, no. 2. Montpellier, France.

Kart, Cary S. 1997. *The realities of aging: An introduction to gerontology.* 6th ed. Boston: Allyn and Bacon.

Koopman-Boyden, Peggy. 1993. *New Zealand's aging society: The implications.* Wellington, New Zealand: Daphne Brasell Associates Press.

Koster, J., and J. Prather, eds. 1997. Counting the world's oldest citizens. *Global Aging Report* 2 (1) (Jan./Feb.): 5.

Mui, A. C., N. G. Choi, and A. Monk. 1998. *Long-term care and ethnicity.* Westport, Conn.: Auburn House.

Nusselder, W. J., K. van der Velden, L. A. van Sonsbeek, M. E. Lenior, and G. van den Bos. 1996. The elimination of selected chronic diseases in a population: The compression and expansion of morbidity. *American Journal of Public Health* 86 (2): 187–88.

Perls, Thomas. 1999. *The living to 100 life expectancy calculator.* On-line: http://www.Livingto100.com

Population Division of the Department for Economic and Social Information and Policy Analysis (UNPD-DESIPA). 1997. *World demographic trends: Report of the secretary general.* Summary of the Thirteenth Session of the Commission on Population and Development. February, New York: United Nations.

Rhee, Seon-Ja. 1995. Health status of elderly Koreans. In *Aging in Korea: Today and tomorrow,* edited by Sung-Jae Choi and Hye-Kyung Suh. Seoul, Korea: Chung-Ang Aptitude Publisher.

Rhoades, E. R., A. J. D'Angelo, and W. B. Hurlburt. 1987. The Indian Health Service record of achievement. *Public Health Reports* 102 (4): 356–60.

Riley, James C. 1990. Long term morbidity and mentality trends: Inverse transition. In *What we know about health transition: The cultural, social, and behavioural determinants of health,* edited by S. C. Caldwell et al., vol.1, 165–88. Canberra: Australian National University.

United Nations Department of International Economic and Social Affairs (UNDIESA). 1991. *World Population Prospects 1990.* ST/ESA/SER.A/122.

U.S. Bureau of the Census. 1996. *Current Population Reports, Special Studies, 65+ in the United States.* Washington, D.C.: GPO.

U.S. Bureau of the Census, International Population Reports. 1992. *An Aging World II.* Washington, D.C.: GPO.

Verbugge, L. M. 1990. The iceberg of disability. In *The legacy of longevity: Health and health care in later life,* edited by S. M. Stahl. Newbury Park, Calif.: Sage.

Zaldivar, R. A. 1998. Health beyond black and white: Asians, Indians, and Hispanics encounter different obstacles. *Detroit Free Press* (Aug. 3). On-line: http://www.freep.com/news/health/qasian3.htm

CHAPTER FOUR

Longevity

While the previous chapter presented demographics regarding the increase in life expectancy around the world, this chapter focuses on factors that contribute to long life (longevity) and theories of longevity. Who lives longer and why? In gerontological studies, biological and sociological theories attempt to explain why some people live longer than other people. Global longevity is attributed to improved nutrition, advances in medical technology, universal health care, healthier diets, a decrease in smoking, better education, higher incomes, and a decrease in life-threatening diseases such as pneumonia, influenza, stroke, and some types of cancer.

In the quest for the fountain of youth, or immortality, the answers are sought in both religion and science. Gerontologists search for the key to longevity in biology, medicine, genetics, immunology, neurology, endocrinology, and pathology. Clues are found in genetics, food/caloric restriction, exercise, lifestyle and behavior studies, and psychoneuroimmunology. Finch defines aging as "a nondescript colloquialism that can mean any change over time, whether during development, young adult life, or senescence. Aging changes may be good (acquisition of wisdom); of no consequence to vitality or morality risk (male pattern baldness); or adverse (arteriosclerosis)" (1990, 671). Biologists debate why the body ages; psychologists try to explain the role of personality and behavior on the aging process; sociologists explore the social environment. Gerontologists are working to put together the pieces to the puzzle of the aging.

Scientists agree that while life expectancy has increased, the human life span has not been extended beyond 121 years. Jean Calment, a French woman, died in 1997 at 121 years old. She was the only person documented to live beyond the 120-year maximum life span. A man in Japan was reported to be 120 years and 237 days when he died (Schulz-Aellen 1997). Scientists predict that living to be 130 years or 135 years will be possible in the not-too-distant future. In 2000, at least 72,000

Americans passed their one-hundredth birthday. It seems likely that one of them will survive to extremely old age. In another forty or fifty years, 1.5 million persons will be centenarians and another 4 or 5 million persons will be 95 years or older. Manton and Stallard (1996) estimate that the number of people ages 85 and older will reach 20 to 25 million in forty or fifty years.

Average life expectancy refers to the average number of years a person can expect to live out of all individuals born at that time. Population mortality is a major determinant of maximum life span. The average mortality rate, or AMR, is an accurate estimate of the rate of senescence. The *rate of senescence* is the rate of deterioration of the biological functions of the species. Finch (1990, 678) defines senescence as "a deteriorative change that causes increased mortality." Finch examines the presumption that age-related changes in organisms are negative and that components of an organism should decay as the end of the life span approaches.

The rate of senescence for humans can be affected by social factors such as social conflicts, malnutrition, or infectious diseases. Thus, the rate of senescence of humans, or the aging of an individual in a certain society, is influenced by social factors in that culture. If the rate of mortality is high, the rate of senescence is low. Humans cannot be expected to reach older ages when the rate of mortality in a country is high. For example, the rate of senescence is low in countries such as Rwanda because the rate of infant mortality is high.

A well-known method for calculating senescence is the Gompertz Model (1825), which is used to determine mortality rates and life span. It has been a major mortality-rate model in gerontology for 60 years. According to Finch, Benjamin Gompertz found that the number of living cells increased in arithmetical progression and decreased in geometrical progression. With this model we conclude that the mortality rate accelerates with age in most populations that live long enough to show senescence but humans have not reached their theoretical life span since the average life span, or average years of life expectancy (about 76 years), has not achieved its potential of 120 years (1990, 13). Buffon, an eighteenth-century biologist, claimed that animals lived six times the period needed to complete their growth. For humans, skeletal maturity is about 20 years; thus, the projected life span is about 120 years (Schulz-Aellen 1997). Cutler (1984) concluded that life span was related to several factors such as rate of development, length of the reproductive cycle, maximum consumption of calories, and size of the brain. He estimated that the potential life span for man was about 115 to 120 years. Thus, scientists seem to agree that the life span has not and will not exceed 120 years.

Maximum life span must be distinguished from life expectancy. *Maximum life span* refers to a biologically determined life span for cells that comprise the organism. It is estimated that, if all diseases were eliminated, humans would probably not live much beyond 120 years (Hooyman and Kiyak 1996). Maximum life span refers to the years that the human species has been documented to survive.

Life span refers to the longevity of long-lived persons or the extreme limit of human longevity, the age beyond which no one can expect to live (Kart 1997). Kart describes the term "prolongevity." Proponents of "prolongevity" believe that human life should be lengthened indefinitely (Kart 1997). Although there have been reports of mountain people in Pakistan and individuals in the former Soviet Union who lived to be 120, 130, or even 150, these claims have not been validated. Russian gerontologist Medevdev offers the following claim of super-longevity:

> The famous man from Yakutia, who was found during the 1959 census to be 130 years old, received especially great publicity because he lived in the place with the terrible climate. When a picture of this outstanding man was published in the central government newspaper, *Isvestia*, the puzzle was quickly solved. A letter was received from a group of Ukrainian villagers who recognized this centenarian as a fellow villager who deserted from the army during the First World War and forged his father's documents. It was found that this man was only 78 years old (Kart 1997, 103).

Why the Body Ages

Scientists, worldwide, study factors influencing the rate of senescence. Documented proof exists that specific factors influence longevity. The life span of humans has not been extended in spite of the increases in life expectancy. The cases of men and women who live to be 120 years are rare. Very few people reach the maximum life span of 120 years because of the cellular changes that disturb equilibrium in the physiological systems. The elderly are vulnerable to diseases due to deterioration of normal homeostasis. Finch (1990) argues that a decline in homeostasis is the major cause of mortality and that, if all diseases were eliminated, about ten years would be added to life expectancy.

Can life be prolonged? The answer has been sought since ancient times and in many civilizations. Can aging be delayed? The ultimate goal is to postpone disease or to remain disease-free for a longer time. Researchers argue how to postpone death and maintain health. Influencing factors are diet, exercise, smoking, alcohol, vitamins, as well as psychological and social factors (stress and coping mechanisms).

Physiological changes over time are visible in hair, skin, face, and body shape. With age, physiological changes occur in internal organs. Changes in cognitive processes are evident with age. The body's capacity to adapt to internal and external demands is lessened. Schulz-Aellen (1997) explains the depletion of functional reserves causing an overall fragility that can lead to death in the absence of disease, a condition called *apocrypha*.

With age, the major functional systems such as the neurological, the cardiovascular, and the pulmonary systems respond with diminished capacity to internal and external demands so that the equilibrium of these systems is disturbed. From the Baltimore Longitudinal Study on Aging, researchers studied the aging of individuals who were disease-free and who ranged in age from 19 to 93 years. From repeated studies, changes were found in the pulmonary, renal, and cardiovascular functions of these persons.

With age the skin changes, the dermis loses collagen and elastin, and the loss of muscle mass increases the tendency of the skin to wrinkle. Older persons have visible aging pigments (melanin) and thinning of the skin. Bones show a decrease in total bone mass, which when severe is osteoporosis. Studies agree that the loss of estrogen contributes to bone loss and the replacement of estrogen is important in bone renewal (Schulz-Aellen 1997).

Changes in biological rhythms are a significant factor in aging. Scientists believe that the loss of synchrony in biological rhythms is responsible for aging (Schulz-Aellen 1997). Disturbances in the normal patterns of sleep are a problem found among elderly people; increased wakefulness during the sleep phase and increased napping during the daytime phase is found to be age-related (Schulz-Aellen 1997).

Table 4.1 illustrates some of the extremes of life spans found among plants and animals. We continue to use animals to study aging and search for indicators of long life.

Genetics

While heredity impacts longevity, it is only one of the factors that contribute to a long life. Personality, social class, relationships, marriage, and stress have predictive value, and studies report a causal relationship between these factors and long life (Schulz-Aellen 1997).

Studies of twins and adopted children provide information. An individual with long-living parents can expect to live a longer life. Studies of adopted children found that children whose biological parents died early of non-accidental diseases were twice as likely to die of non-accidental diseases. Males have a 10% to 20% shorter life span than

Table 4.1 Life Spans of Plants and Animals

Plant or Animal	Age (In Years)
Octopus	3–4 years
Rat	4–5 years
Earthworm	more than 6 years
Rabbit	10–13 years
Tarantula	15 years
Bear	40 years
Chimpanzee	45 years
Frog	1–60 years
Alligator	50–60 years
African Elephant	more than 70 years
Human	120 years
Lake Sturgeon	more than 150 years
Trees (Sequoia)	5,000 years

Source: Schulz-Aellen, 1997

females in many mammalian species. The shorter life span has been attributed to the Y chromosome. The likelihood that male sexual hormones reduce life span was noted by the observation that eunuchs live somewhat longer than normal men (Schulz-Aellen 1997).

Monozygotic (identical) twin studies found that they die within three years of each other, while the life span of dizygotic (fraternal) twins varies by about six years. Twins inherit specific genes that may set limits on their longevity through predisposition to particular diseases such as atherosclerosis, cancer, etc. Twins may possess similar responses to the management of stress, in personality traits, and other behavioral responses.

A startling genetic finding is the association of apolipoprotein E (ApoE4) with Alzheimer's disease. Possession of the ApoE4 gene is a strong predictor of Alzheimer's disease. Genetic connections are in the occurrence of cardiovascular disease, ischemic heart disease, lower cholesterol levels, fragile X syndrome, and several other diseases. Genetic engineering and gene therapy are powerful methods to prevent age-related disorders. However, it is not yet possible to alter death genes and increase life span. Study of the genome is the total inventory of heritable nucleic acids, including DNA, which affect the human being. Genetic studies are providing valuable information about longevity.

The Role of Personality and Lifestyle Behaviors

Personality characteristics influence the ability to manage stress and cope with life's situations and the behaviors that are health-seeking or health-damaging (Schulz-Aellen 1997). Reaction to the stresses of the environment profoundly affect health. There is some evidence that cancer is related to tension and feelings of helplessness (Schulz-Aellen 1997).

There is evidence that personality characteristics determine the manner in which people age. For example, what type of personality has greater levels of activity, or satisfactory coping mechanisms for accepting illness or aging-related physical changes? Centenarians are reported to have a positive outlook and a sense of optimism (Poon et al. 1992).

Health is linked to life satisfaction and well-being. People who have good health are happier, have a better sense of well-being, have friends, and tend to be satisfied with life. Evidence exists that depression

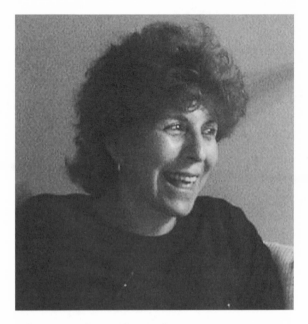

A happy attitude contributes to longevity.

produces a defective biological environment that leads to the emergence of diseases (Schulz-Aellen 1997).

Happiness has been found to be related to marital status. Generally, married persons are happier than single persons, particularly men. In a cross-national study in the United States, Western Europe, Japan, Taiwan, and several other Asian countries, researchers found the average rate of death for single men and women was twice that of married men and women. The greatest difference was at ages 25 to 44 years. Sharing of life situations seems to positively influence physical and mental health.

Stress is considered to have pathogenic features. In 1936, Hans Seyle reported that chronic stressors caused peptic ulcers and immune deficiencies (Schulz-Aellen 1997). A stressor is defined as a perturbation in the outside world that disrupts homeostasis. Stressors produce varied biological responses that affect the adrenal system, the immunological system, and the neurological system. Stress-related disorders include myopathy, fatigue, diabetes, stress-induced hypertension, digestive ulcers, amenorrhea, impotency, loss of libido, and neuronal death.

Scientific evidence links stress to disease (Schulz-Aellen 1997). However, it is difficult to prove a causal relationship between stress and disease. There is no evidence that stress can cause a tumor. Aging is observed to decrease the capacity to respond to stressors due to a less efficient regulation of homeostasis. Chronic stress is believed to accelerate neuronal degeneration during aging. Negative effects of stress on the immune system seem to be the activity of natural killer cells and may, as a consequence, cause a person to be more susceptible to disease.

The role of the immune system is to protect against invading microorganisms. A developing field of science, called psychoneuroimmunology, is examining the impact of the social environment and stress on the neuro-endocrine-immune system. Psychoneuroimmunologists study how psychological factors influence disease development and the epidemiology of diseases such as in the etiology of cancer.

A healthy diet, exercise, vitamins, avoiding stress, avoiding smoking and alcohol, and a positive outlook are related to longevity. Gerontologists argue whether living longer and healthier lives is related to nutrition and exercise. So-called life-extension products such as special diets, megadoses of vitamins, and herb supplements are trends that are creating new businesses. Scientists agree that lifestyle habits such as exercise and balanced nutrition improve the quality of life and may prolong life, while other habits such as smoking or alcohol abuse may shorten life (National Institute on Aging 1993). Physical activity and its relationship to health are important subjects of study; exercise physiologists are concerned with these issues.

Among adults ages 35 and older, heart disease is the leading cause of death in developed countries (U.S. Bureau of the Census, International Population Reports 1992). Deaths from cancers rank a close second. In North America, death rates from heart disease peaked in the 1960s and since then have declined by almost 50%. France, the United Kingdom, Belgium, Finland, and the Netherlands report heart disease mortality declines of 10% to 20%. In Greece, Yugoslavia, and several Eastern European nations, heart disease mortality increased from 20% to 40% for men from the 1960s to the 1980s. In the United States in 1990, heart disease and cancer were equally prevalent, each accounting for one-third of all deaths in the age group of 65 to 74 years (U.S. Bureau of the Census, International Population Reports 1992).

Cardiovascular scientists worldwide study the influence of diet and exercise on heart disease. These studies have led to improvements in the rate of disabilities from falls, strokes, heart disease, vision and hearing losses, and mobility problems.

Diet plays a vital role throughout the life span. Obesity is associated with greater morbidity. Obesity increases the incidence of diseases such as diabetes, hypertension, stroke, and cardiovascular diseases (National Institute on Aging 1993). Nutrition influences bodily functions such as gastrointestinal functions, immune function, and even cognitive abilities; nutrition is associated with osteoporosis, cancer, and even infectious diseases such as tuberculosis. Dietary recommendations to reduce the risk of heart disease are:

❖ Reduce fat intake to 30% of calories a day.
❖ Reduce the intake of cholesterol to less than 300 milligrams a day.
❖ Eat at least five combinations daily of vegetables and fruits.
❖ Maintain protein intake at moderate levels.
❖ Limit total daily intake of salt to 6 grams or less.

(National Institute on Aging 1993)

Dietary changes improve health by lowering cholesterol levels, lowering blood pressure, and decreasing the risk of heart disease and susceptibility to some types of cancers. A quite controversial dietary recommendation is the result of food restriction studies, or FR studies. Strong evidence exists regarding the effects of FR in animals (rats and monkeys), but there are few studies in humans (National Institute on Aging 1993).

Food Restriction/Caloric Restriction

Food restriction (FR), or caloric restriction as it is also known, demonstrates evidence for extension of the life span in animal species (Schulz-Aellen 1997). There is evidence that age-related diseases are retarded by FR, which induces changes in cell membranes, delays the progression of immune deficiency with age, and protects and maintains cellular homeostasis. In humans, the effects of FR on longevity are unknown. However, people with particular diets that are maintained for religious reasons or who maintain specific diets (vegetarians), and those who, for religious reasons, abstain from alcohol, coffee, and tobacco are found to have higher longevity.

Caloric restriction alters the rate of aging in animals. Reducing food intake lowers the animal's metabolic rate and slows aging (National Institute on Aging 1993). The exact mechanism by which caloric restriction increases survival is not known. At this time, there is little evidence that caloric restriction can change the life span for humans. The only data available suggest a relationship between weight and longevity. Data indicate that people at the two extremes of weight have the shortest life spans. In the mice study, calories were restricted and the obese mice outlived the normal mice on normal diets despite the fact that they were still overweight (National Institute on Aging 1993). New studies are under way on the effect of long-term caloric restriction on aging monkeys (DeLany et al. 1999), and the effects of lifelong moderate caloric restriction remain unclear for human survival (McShane, Wilson, and Wise 1999).

Vitamins

Vitamin supplements enhance the nutritional needs of older persons who have poor eating patterns or who are unable to maintain good nutritional intake. Evidence exists that the vitamin needs of older persons may be greater than that of younger persons; however, there is also widespread misuse of vitamins. Vitamins may offer some possible benefits, but this remains an area of medicine with little scientific study.

The benefits of vitamin A reportedly include preventing night blindness; retarding macular degeneration; and reducing the risk of breast, lung, colon, and prostate cancer (Schulz-Aellen 1997). Vitamin B_1 (thiamin) is necessary for the normal functioning of all cells, especially the nerve cells. Vitamin B_2 (riboflavin) is needed for the production of certain hormones and the formation of red blood cells. Vitamin B_{12} is essential for nerve cells, and a deficiency can manifest itself clinically with disorientation, moodiness, agitation, and hallucinations. Researchers found that vitamin deficiencies are associated with dementia, depression, or psychosis (Schulz-Aellen 1997).

Vitamin C has a powerful antioxidant action and plays an important role in the metabolism of cholesterol and the repair of tissue damage. Vitamin D is essential in preventing breast cancer, prostate cancer, and colon cancer. Vitamin E affects the immune system and acts as a powerful antioxidant. Vitamin K may play a role in the prevention of cancer and osteoporosis. Calcium is recommended for the prevention of osteoporosis (Schulz-Aellen 1997).

Aspirin is an anti-inflammatory drug that decreases the tendency of blood platelets to aggregate in certain vessels. In 1994, Solomon and Hart reported that aspirin is beneficial for myocardial infarction, transient ischemic heart attacks, unstable angina, and stroke (Schulz-Aellen 1997). The U.S. Preventive Services Task Force recommends low doses of aspirin every day for men older than 50 years for the prevention of myocardial infarction. Woods (1994) suggests that only those women who have a high risk of heart disease should take aspirin because the risk benefits may be different in women, and studies are inconclusive for women. Before taking aspirin, it is recommended that one consult a physician.

Exercise

The older person of today is unlike the older person of yesterday, and the older person of tomorrow will be different from the older person of today. This cohort of older persons is healthier and more active. A decade ago it was rare for an 80-year-old person to run in a marathon or to skydive.

Lack of exercise and physical inactivity are linked to cardiovascular problems, high-density lipoprotein (HDL) levels, loss of muscle mass, glucose intolerance, and stroke. Exercise triggers physiological changes that are beneficial to the body's functions. Aging brings about a decline in cardiovascular functions and muscle mass in older persons, but exercise positively affects these functions. Exercise positively influences hypertension, which is reported to be a common health risk for individuals older than 65 years (Schulz-Aellen 1997). Scientists found that endurance exercise training lowers blood pressure in cases of moderate hypertension.

Exercise affects glucose tolerance. As many as 40% of persons older than 65 have undiagnosed diabetes (Schulz-Aellen 1997). Aerobic exercise is associated with better glucose tolerance in older persons. Vigorous exercise for at least 30 to 45 minutes every other day is recommended to maintain normal glucose and insulin metabolism (Schulz-Aellen 1997).

Exercise has positive effects on hyperlipidemia. Persons with heart disease tend to have high levels of LDL-C (bad cholesterol) and low levels of HDL-C (good cholesterol). Physical training improves the regulation of lipid metabolism. Osteoporosis affects about 50% of older women and 25% of older men. Osteoporosis is responsible for bone loss and fracture. Bone loss can be reduced and even restored by increased exercise. Postmenopausal women who exercise regularly can gain bone mass (Schulz-Aellen 1997). Finally, exercise has been shown to affect mood. Physical activity stimulates the synthesis of endorphins, which produces a feeling of well-being. Recommendations from the 1995 Blair Study of 27,000 men indicate that longevity is associated with vigorous physical activity (Schulz-Aellen 1997). (See Appendix B for a quiz on bone loss.)

Smoking and Alcohol Use

Because tobacco is considered a life-shortening drug, smoking is a major health hazard. Smoking accounts for 80% of all lung cancers, 25% of all heart attacks, and 80% of bronchitis and emphysema cases. Tobacco affects disturbances in metabolism, especially the lipoproteins. Smoking is currently an epidemic in Asian countries, especially China. Smoking in China is rampant and, as a result, about 50 million Chinese now under the age of 20 will die of tobacco-related diseases (Schulz-Aellen 1997).

Alcohol consumption affects the nervous system, and its impact on longevity is receiving more attention. Sharper and his colleagues in 1988 suggested that moderate drinkers have a lower rate of mortality from cardiovascular diseases (Schulz-Aellen 1997). Not all scientists support the view that one glass of wine a day is helpful in preventing heart disease (Schulz-Aellen 1997).

Summary

Longevity is the search for the fountain of youth and immortality. The factors that contribute to long, healthy lives are under global study and have been sought for centuries. Genetics, diet (less food), nutrition, exercise, and lifestyle habits (avoiding alcohol or smoking) are subjects of exploration. Personality and behaviors (stress management and happiness) may be influencing factors that contribute to long life. The answers to the puzzle of aging are yet not completely understood.

References

Cutler, R. G. 1984. Evolutionary biology of aging and longevity in mammalian species. In *Aging and cell function,* edited by J. E. Johnson Jr. New York: Plenum.

DeLany, J., B. Hansen, N. Bodkin, J. Hannah, and G. Bray. 1999. Long-term calorie restriction reduces energy expenditure in aging monkeys. *Journal of Gerontology: Biological Sciences* 54A (1): B5–B11.

Finch, C. E. 1990. *Longevity, senescence, and the genome.* Chicago and London: University of Chicago Press.

Hooyman, N., and H. A. Kiyak. 1996. *Social gerontology: A multidisciplinary perspective.* 4th ed. Boston: Allyn and Bacon.

Kart, Cary S. 1997. *The realities of aging: An introduction to gerontology.* 6th ed. Boston: Allyn and Bacon.

Manton, Kenneth, and Eric Stallard. 1996. Age limit pegged at 130+. *Brown University Long-Term Care Quality Advisor* 8 (18): 7–8. Electronic reference: University of South Carolina Infotrac, Health Reference Center—Academic.

McShane, T., M. Wilson, and P. Wise. 1999. Effects of lifelong moderate caloric restriction on levels or neuropeptide Y, proopiomelanocortin, and galanin mRNA. *Journal of Gerontology: Biological Sciences* 54A (1): B14–B21.

National Institute on Aging. 1993. *Answers about: The aging woman and the aging man.* Washington, D.C.: U.S. Department of Health and Human Services, Public Health Service, and National Institutes of Health.

Poon, L. W., G. M. Clayton, P. Martin, M. A. Johnson, B. C. Courtenay, A. L. Sweaney, S. B. Merriam, B. S. Pless, and S. B. Thielman. 1992. *The Georgia centenarian study.* Amityville, N.Y.: Baywood.

Schulz-Aellen, Marie-Francoise. 1997. *Aging and human longevity.* Boston: Birkhauser Boston.

U.S. Bureau of the Census, International Population Reports. 1992. *An Aging World II.* P25, 92–3. Washington, D.C.: GPO.

U.S. Bureau of Census, Statistical Abstracts. 1996. *Current Population Reports, Special Studies. P23–190, 65+ in the United States.* Washington, D.C.: GPO.

Woods, S. E. 1994. Primary prevention of coronary heart disease in women. *Archives of Family Medicine* 3: 361–64.

CHAPTER FIVE

A Biopsychosocial Perspective of Aging

Gerontology is a multidisciplinary field of study, and its practice requires a biopsychosocial perspective. This chapter presents an overview of select biological theories of aging, psychological perspectives, and social gerontological issues that influence the lives of older adults. Working with older adults requires specialized knowledge of the influences of health and psychological state and social environment.

Biological theories explore why the body ages and dies. Scientists study biological theories including the wear-and-tear theory, the autoimmune theory, and the cell theory. Psychological studies explore behavior in late life including studies of attitudes, learning, memory, intellectual abilities, motivation, emotions, personality, and social relationships. In social gerontology, selected topics are families, sexuality, social supports, living arrangements, religion, and social issues.

Biological Theories of Aging

Biological theories of aging endeavor to explain the body's aging process. Scientists explore whether aging has a single cause or multiple causes. Why does the body age? Currently, no single theory of aging explains all of the complexities of the body's aging process. If the body's aging complexities are understood, interventions may be possible to delay or to halt aging.

Theories of aging fall into two groups: "programmed" theories and error theories. The programmed theories argue that aging follows a biological timetable. Programmed theories include theories such as programmed senescence, the endocrine theory, and the immunological theory. *Programmed senescence* argues that aging is a result of the sequential switching on and off of certain genes, with senescence being defined as the time when age-associated deficits are manifested. *Endocrine theory* proposes that hormones control the pace of aging. *Immunological theory* proposes that a programmed decline in the immune system function leads to increased vulnerability to infectious disease, aging, and death. These theoretical perspectives argue that aging and death are genetically programmed, that there is an order to the predictable changes of the body, and that an aging and death clock is located in the DNA of each cell. Hayflick argues that each species has a fixed life span, an idea which supports the belief that some sort of programming must be involved in aging and death (Belsky 1990).

The immune system is described as an aging clock that protects against disease by producing cells that can fight off invader cells. A strong immune system eliminates foreign substances, but in a weak immune system deficiencies hinder the body's ability to fight off illnesses. Deficiencies in the immune system's ability to recognize its own cells may cause it to attack its own tissues and create an autoimmune response. This response may be partly responsible for age-related diseases such as dementia and diabetes.

Error Theories

Damage, or error, theories suggest that environmental assaults to our systems gradually lead to deterioration and dysfunction. The *error theories* include the wear-and-tear theory, rate-of-living theory, cross-linking, free radical theory, cellular theory, error catastrophe theory, and somatic mutation theory.

Wear and Tear

The *wear-and-tear theory* proposes that cells and tissues wear out just as a car does after a great deal of use. Aging is the result of deterioration of the organs necessary for living. This theory explains why parts of the body become worn or frail over time, such occurs as in bone loss, cataracts, heart changes, etc. Transplants and surgical repair of organs may help to prolong life, as in heart or kidney transplants and cataract surgery for vision loss. Parts replacement and surgical repair may not prolong life but can enhance life. Weismann, a biogerontologist writing in 1882, is responsible for the wear-and-tear theory. He discovered that there are two kinds of cells: germ cells, which never die, and somatic cells, which die. He argued that aging takes place because somatic cells cannot renew themselves and so, after wear and tear, they die (Moody 1994). However, there is no evidence that hard work on the body will shorten life. In contrast, there is evidence that appropriate exercise can reduce some of the effects of aging.

Rate-of-Living Theory

The *rate-of-living theory* argues that the greater an organism's rate of oxygen basal metabolism the shorter its life span, and that the ability to maintain homeostasis is slower in older persons. Stress and body changes from medication and changes in the body's ability to regulate temperatures are evidence that the self-regulating mechanisms of the body decrease with age.

Cross-Linking

Cross-linking refers to the belief that an accumulation of cross-linked proteins damages cells and tissues. According to this theory, changes in the elasticity of some parts of the body, such as skin and the lens of the eye, are a result of the accumulation of cross-linking compounds. Cross-linking may be caused by free radicals.

Free Radical Theory

The *free radical theory* speculates that oxygen radicals cause cells and organs to stop functioning and to accumulate damage. Free radicals are reactive chemicals produced randomly during normal metabolism. These biochemicals produce cellular damage and impair the organism's ability to function. Free radicals are evident in emphysema, arteriosclerosis, cancer, arthritis, cirrhosis, and diabetes. According to this theory, damage caused by free radicals contributes to aging.

Cellular Theory

In 1961, Hayflick reported that cells reproduce a programmed number of times and then die. Cells develop for about 30 years and then "coast" for a maximum of 75 years (Kimmel 1990). Hayflick and his associates discovered that normal human cells go through a finite number of divisions and then stop reproducing. The maximum numbers of divisions are known as the *Hayflick limit*. Hayflick found that if cells are taken from fetal tissue they replicate about 100 times, but if they are taken from a 70-year-old they replicate only about 20 or 30 times (Moody 1994). A genetic code is responsible for the finite capability of cells to reproduce, and the cellular limit is related to the maximum life span of the species.

Error Catastrophe Theory

Damage to mechanisms that synthesize proteins results in the accumulation of faulty proteins to catastrophic levels, which damage cells, tissues, and organs—a process known as the Random Damage Theory (Belsky 1990). According to this theory, accumulating mistakes in the cell's ability to produce proteins are the main cause of aging and death (Belsky 1990).

Somatic Mutation Theory

This theory proposes that genetic mutations occur and accumulate with increasing age, causing cells to deteriorate and malfunction (National Institute of Health 1993).

Kimmel defines physiological aging as "a decline in physiological competence that inevitably increases the incidence and intensifies the effects of accidents, disease, and other forms of environmental stress" (1990, 346). Theorists agree that there is no single cause of aging (Kimmel 1990). The loss of physical functioning is not debatable but the cause is yet undetermined.

An interesting mythological story tells a tale of a woman who asked the gods for one wish—immortality for her lover. The gods asked if she had any other wishes and she answered no, this one wish was all she wanted. Tholnious, her lover, was granted immortality. Later, she realized that she had forgotten to ask for good health for him. So Tholnious aged and became increasingly frail and weak until he was as small and feeble as a cricket, but he would never die. Immortality may not be a blessing (Dychtwald 1995).

Since the 1970s there has been an explosion of research in the field of aging, especially in cellular biology, molecular biology, and neurobiology of aging, the study of the aging brain. The *Handbook of the Biology of Aging,* edited by Schneider and Rowe (1996), is an important source for more extensive material on the biology of aging. This chapter presents an overview of essential information.

Psychology of Aging

Psychology is defined by France as "the systematic study of behavior and factors that influence behavior" (1990, 87). Psychology of aging is the study of factors that influence behavior in late life. Geropsychologists study motivation, memory, sensory behavior, learning, intelligence, and personality. Mental illness and mental health will be discussed in another chapter of this book. Included here are topics that are crucial to understanding the behaviors of older adults, including personality, cognition, and intelligence. The reader can find comprehensive material in texts such as Belsky's *The Psychology of Aging: Theory, Research, and Interventions* (1990) and Birren and Schaie's *Handbook of the Psychology of Aging* (1996).

Birren and Birren (1990) present an overview of the history and development of psychological knowledge. Until recently, psychology ignored aging and adult development. One of the earliest books on the psychology of aging, published in 1922, was G. S. Hall's review of the knowledge of aging acquired at that period, *Senescence: The Second Half of Life*. Another early book was Cowdry's *Problems of Aging*, published in 1939 (Birren and Schoots 1996).

Intelligence

Evidence is found to support the belief that intelligence remains stable throughout the life cycle. Longitudinal-designed studies did not find significant declines in intellectual ability until a person is older than 60 years (France 1990), and most declines occur later, at 65 or 70 years. Decline refers to general intelligence, which includes specific skills (information processing, memory, attention, and cognitive structure). Researchers distinguish between fluid intelligence and crystallized intelligence (Belsky 1990).

Fluid intelligence describes task performance not influenced by level of education, including response speed, attention span, and immediate reasoning ability. Fluid intelligence is dependent on the efficient functioning of the central nervous system. Fluid abilities begin to decline after the age of 14. Speed task performance begins to decline in early adult years. Fluid intelligence is associated with physiology (France 1990).

Crystallized intelligence is heavily influenced by education and socialization (vocabulary, associations, and technical skills), and it is described as the store of knowledge accumulated over time (Belsky 1990). While fluid intelligence declines, crystallized intelligence increases throughout adulthood. A decline in fluid, speeded, and performance intellectual skills but an increase in crystallized unspeeded and verbal intellectual skills is evident in adulthood (France 1990).

The fluid/crystallized dichotomy seems to fit real-life phenomena. Philosophers, historians, or writers reach their peak later in life than do people in professions that demand totally novel ways to solve problems. While age is more of an enemy to air traffic controllers, who must quickly analyze data, it is more of an advantage to the executive who depends on experience to make decisions (Belsky 1990).

An interesting study by Sward, in 1945, compared old and young professors and found that professors, aged 60 to 80 years, surpassed their 30-year-old colleagues on vocabulary and information tests (Belsky 1990). Consistently, when test content is related to experience, such as vocabulary tests, older persons do better than younger persons. Experience with educationally related material seems to make a significant difference in performance.

Schaie (1996) reviewed research on mental abilities and reported little decline in age-related mental abilities. Decline in mental abilities affected less than one-third of the participants until age 74, and by age 81 only between 30% and 40% were affected. Decline in psychological competence occurs in most persons as the 80s and 90s approach and much of the loss is experienced in challenging, complex, or stressful situations. Cohort studies report marked improvement in performance with successive generations due to improved nutrition, health status, increased educational opportunities, and the conquest of childhood diseases. In a fourteen-year study, significant intellectual decline was noted in a group of persons with cardiovascular disease (Schaie 1996).

Evidence exists of age-related decline in learning speed. However, questions remain. Although there is change in reaction time and decrease in fluid abilities with age, there are data that crystallized abilities may increase in later life and that some variables affect the rate of decline, including levels of education, income, occupational status, intact marriage, and even lengthy marriage to an intelligent spouse (Schaie 1996).

Cognition and Memory
Cognition is defined as "the process of knowing in the broadest sense, including memory, perception, judgment, etc." (Geralnik 1974). A primary complaint and concern of older persons is memory loss. Memory

loss is feared because it is associated with early stages of Alzheimer's disease. Salthouse defines cognitive competence as "the utilization of one's abilities—cognitive, interpersonal, and others—in adapting to particular situations" (1990, 311). From this perspective, cognitive ability and cognitive competence are at least somewhat independent because it is possible for a person with a low level of cognitive ability to achieve a high degree of competence by maximizing available abilities for functioning.

Memory studies, including studies of short-term memory or working memory, show little age-related decline unless the activities require active manipulation of the information or division of attention. Psychological research includes studies of memory with meaningful material. Retrieval seems to become slower with age but, if cued, information comes readily. Distraction during the storing process can interfere with the information processed and can affect retrieval of information. Whereas there is evidence of decline in specific skills, well-practiced, familiar, and adaptive skills are retained into old age (France 1990). Older people perform best when the memory task is relevant to their lives (Belsky 1990). In a study using age-relevant words such as retirement and widowhood, older people outperformed younger people (Belsky 1990). Rodin and Langer filmed three actors, ages 20, 50, and 70 years, who read the same speech. In the monologue the actors referred to memory lapses such as, "I forgot my keys." Older people who saw the film were just as likely as the younger people to describe the 70-year-old as mentally deteriorating (Belsky 1990). Normal forgetting in older persons is exaggerated and interpreted as a sign of aging or disease.

Personality Theories

Personality refers to stable, distinctive patterns of behavior, thought, and emotion that characterize a person's adaptation to the situations of life (France 1990). Personality characteristics are reportedly stable from young adulthood to old age among healthy, community-dwelling older adults (France 1990). Personality stability is described as the hallmark of adult development. Personality is determined in the first five years of life. Years do not change the personality. Personality studies continue in two directions—trait models and developmental models. McCrae and Costa describe a five-factor model of personality as follows:

1. Neuroticism is a tendency toward maladjustment (anxiety, depression, hostility, and emotional distress) rather than mental health.

2. Extroversion reflects outgoingness, warmth, and gregariousness.

3. Openness to experience involves willingness to take risks, to try new things.

4. Agreeableness.

5. Conscientiousness.

(Belsky 1990)

Costa argues that happiness is an enduring aspect of personality. A happy 25-year-old will most likely be a happy, stable older person while a cranky, miserable old person was once a cranky young adult. However, even Costa points out that some older people do change radically over the years (Belsky 1990). Dimensions of personality such as introversion and extroversion were described by Neugarten, Havighurst, and Tobin (1968).

From developmental models of personality, theorists argue about patterns of continued cognitive development in adulthood. Erikson's theory of personality development includes eight stages of ego development. He stated that the ego had conflict in each stage, and the solution at each stage of ego development had consequences for the next stage. The last stage of ego development was termed ego integrity versus ego despair. In this stage, a person looks back on life and has a sense of wholeness and satisfaction (ego integrity) or despair (ego despair). A person may despair, fear death, and wish for another chance to change life's circumstances. Another person is satisfied with life and is ready for the inevitable.

Peck (1968) divided adult life into two chronological divisions, middle age and old age. He described periods of psychological stages as *ego differentiation* and *work role preoccupation,* and *body transcendence* or *body preoccupation.* Individuals who focus their lives on body aches and pains, or equate pleasure in life with physical well-being, perceive a decline in health or physical vigor as a weakness and are described as being in a state of body preoccupation. An ever-increasing concern with the state of the body is referred to as body preoccupation. On the other hand, those persons who enjoy life in spite of declines in physical health and who define happiness in terms of creative activities and relationships are described as reaching a state of body transcendence. Peck (1968, 91) describes living in this way:

To live so generously and unselfishly that the prospect of personal death—the night of the ego, it might be called—looks and feels less important than the secure knowledge that one has built a broader, longer future than any one ego could ever encompass. Through children, through contributions to the culture, through friendship—these are the ways in which human beings can achieve enduring significance for their actions which goes beyond the limit of their own skins and their own lives. It may, indeed, be the only known kind of self-perpetuation after death.

Levinson's model (1978) pays attention to the relationship of physical changes and personality. He describes the mid-life transition as mid-life crises. Critics of Levinson's study report that he did not include women and that the oldest person in the study was 50 years old (France 1990). Subsequent studies that included women found that women progress through the same developmental periods of early adulthood as do men (Belsky 1990). However, the mid-life crisis stage found in men at age 40 is not definitive. Studies by McCrae and Costa suggest no evidence for the mid-life crisis theory (Belsky 1990).

Loevinger's model is an ego-developmental theory, which describes four stages across the adolescent and adult years: conformist, conscientious, autonomous, and integrated. For additional information, the reader is referred to other sources of psychological research, including extensive material on creativity in aging, psychopathology and mental health in the older adult, psychological interventions, and the use of psychometric assessment tools with the older adult (Belsky 1990).

Social Gerontology

Social gerontology includes research on social aspects and social structures affecting the lives of older persons. Families (older married couples/the blended family, adult children and aging parents, grandparents raising grandchildren), widowhood, employment, retirement, sexuality, social supports, living arrangements, religion and spirituality, and leisure activities require attention.

Families

The family has been romanticized. A nostalgic recollection of the "good old days" brings to mind a time when mom and dad, the children, and

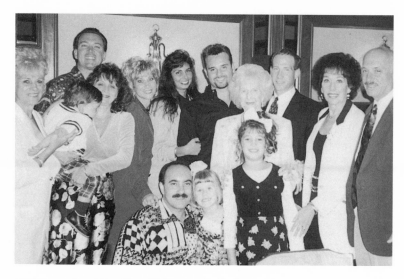

Multigenerational families will increase in the future.

grandparents all lived happily together in the same house. The roman-
tic image extends to remembering that older adults were loved and
respected in the "good old days." Western cultures envy the eastern philosophy of filial responsibility. Added to this nostalgic image are neighborhood changes in urban areas, along with the myth of wonderful
rural neighbors who pitched in and helped provide care in time of
need.

The family image as it has been romanticized disappeared in modern society, a loss which seems to be worldwide. The myth romanticiz-
ing the family and family values is strong and pervades western and
eastern cultures. Positive changes are often ignored in this image. The
structure and roles of families have changed. Although family members
provide the bulk of care for older persons, older adults are portrayed as
being alone and abandoned in nursing homes. This portrayal is untrue
because more than 75% of older adults live in family settings in the
United States, and in Australia more than 90% of older persons live in
families (Moody 1994). Families provide the bulk of care for older family members. Middle-aged women will spend more years taking care of
parents and parents-in-law than caring for children under 18 years
(Moody 1994). In 1979, Shanas, in a cross-national study (United

States, England, and Denmark), found that 80% of care for the frail elderly is provided by families (Moody 1994). This figure has not changed significantly in the 1990s.

A worldwide controversy centers on whether family or government should be responsible for the care of older persons. Singapore's system of parent care requires that adult children set aside a fund for the care of their aged parents. In Chinese cultures, filial piety has included the duty to support parents. This tradition is changing in modern Asia. Modern families include blended families, single-parent families, multigenerational families, immigrant families, childless families, grandparent head-of-household families, and nuclear families.

Older Marriages

Marriages are lasting longer than ever before. Sixty-four percent of couples who married in their early twenties can expect their marriages to

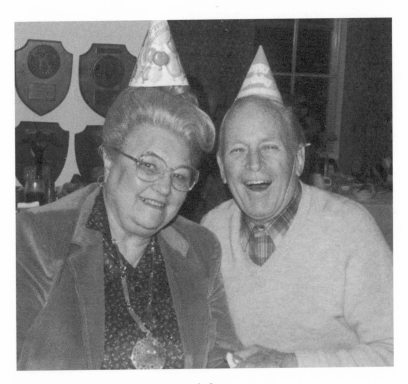

Marriages are lasting longer than ever before.

last about forty years (Belsky 1990). At least one-third of the time will be spent without children, or living in an empty nest (Belsky 1990). In the 1990s couples married later and had children later than was done previously. Evidence exists that older adults are divorcing after twenty-five or thirty years of marriage and are remarrying to create new family relationships of children, stepchildren, grandchildren, and step-grand-children. About 20% of older people are childless (Hooyman and Kiyak 1996). Later marriages suggest a new group of older persons without children who will not have the social support of children and grandchildren but who may have support from friends, neighbors, and church.

Adult Children and Aging Parents

Adult children of aging parents are sometimes referred to as the sand-wich generation since they are in the middle of raising young children and caring for aging parents (Moody 1994). Due to increased years of life, middle-aged adult children are caring for aging parents at a time in their lives when they expected to be free of the responsibility of raising children. Adult children fill the empty nest with aging parents.

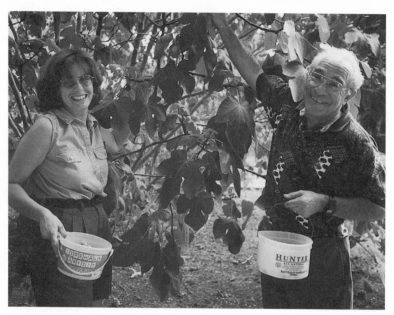

Adult children can enjoy time with their parents.

Shanas, in 1979, dispelled the myth that older adults are abandoned by their children. The study reported that most children live close to their parents, more than three-quarters within a thirty-minute drive; more than half had seen each other that day or the day before; about four in five had visited within the past week. And there was a bond between the adult child and the aging parent (Moody 1994).

Parents want to live near their children but not in the same household. In 1900, more than 60% of persons older than 65 years lived with their adult children. In 1957, one-third of parents shared their children's households; in 1975, this figure was only 19% (Belsky 1990). This trend continues in postmodern societies.

In Europe, multigenerational living arrangements are uncommon. Western societies prefer separate residences for nuclear families. Intimacy at a distance reflects the common desire by older people to live independently away from grown children. This pattern is becoming more popular in Asian societies as economic independence becomes possible for young and old families.

Another American myth is the "Walton family myth," in which a multigenerational household lives together harmoniously. Multigenerational families were rare due to high rates of mortality of older persons. In addition, living together does not always reflect closer relationships (Belsky 1990). Researchers found no relationship between frequency of contact between parents and children and closeness of the generations (Belsky 1990).

Grandparents

Grandparents serve many roles in the lives of their adult children and their grandchildren. Grandparents are described as "family watchdogs" by Troll (Belsky 1990). Grandparents are family mediators who provide financial or emotional support to adult children or grandchildren, serve as links to the past, and in the 1990s grandparents have taken on the role of raising grandchildren.

The topic of grandparenthood is of new interest to gerontology. The functions of grandparenthood have changed due to increased geographic mobility, divorce, employed middle-aged women, retired men, and reconstituted families. Studies on life satisfaction for grandparents found that the role of grandparent is not a primary source of identity,

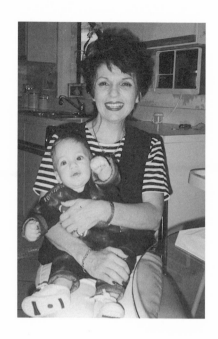

Grandmothers today do not fit the stereotype of grandmothers of just thirty years ago.

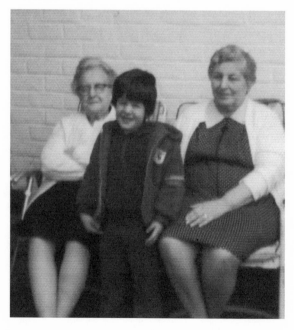

but that friendships and organizational activities appear to be related to life satisfaction (Hooyman and Kiyak 1996).

Grandparents serve a role in providing family continuity. Grand parents derive emotional gratification from their grandchildren. Geographic distance is not necessarily a barrier when a close relationship is established early. Grandparenthood provides opportunities for grandparents to experience feelings of immortality. Grandparent and grandchildren relationships change over time with less contact as grand-children become older. Grandfathers appear to be most closely linked to sons of their sons and grandmothers to daughters of their daughters (Hooyman and Kiyak 1996).

Some grandparents are responsible for the care of their grandchildren due to their children's problems with drugs, poverty, AIDS, incarceration, emotional problems, or criminal offenses, which are growing in numbers in America. About 3 million children live with grandparents without parents present (Hooyman and Kiyak 1996).

The incidence of sole grandparenting has doubled in the last decade. National organizations have formed such as ROCKING (Raising Our Children's Kids: An Intergenerational Network of Grandparenting, Inc.) and the National Coalition of Grandparents (NCOG). In 1997, 780,000 homes in the United States included a grandparent and grandchild without a parent present (Pruncho 1999). Close to half of these households, 47%, are white; 35.9% are African American; and 15.1% are Hispanic. Social-service providers estimate that, in inner cities, somewhere between 30% and 50% of children under 18 years of age live with grandparents. Child maltreatment by the parents is the primary cause of grandparents raising grandchildren.

Grandparents caring for grandchildren are more prevalent in developing countries—more prevalent that might be expected. In Fiji, more than 70% of persons older than 60 years were actively involved in the care of their grandchildren. In South Korea, Malaysia, and the Philippines, the number was about 54%. In Fiji, men and women were equally involved in the care of grandchildren, but in most countries, caregiving grandparents are predominately female. Grandparents play a major role in the upbringing of grandchildren (Tout 1994). Great-grandparenting will become more of the norm with older adults living well into their seventies and eighties. With the growing numbers of grandparents and great-grandparents, it will not be uncommon to see four- and five-generation families.

Widowhood and Divorce

Women continue to outlive men by about seven years and, although the gap is narrowing, two of three women can expect to be widows when they are in their seventies. The loss of a spouse is considered one of life's most stressful events. Remarriage is unlikely for women. In America, the average age of widowhood is 56 years, while average life expectancy is 80 years. Thus, the years of widowhood are more than twenty-five (Hooyman and Kiyak 1996).

The proportion of non-white widows is twice that of white women. Older people may experience a number of losses in addition to the loss of a spouse. Frequently, loss of a spouse necessitates changes in the living environment. Research is inconclusive whether the stress of widowhood is greater for young women than for old women, or if widowhood is more difficult for men or women. Men are better off financially and in terms of remarriage opportunities. However, women form strong social supports for each other.

Economic and social support is important for widows in the Middle East, Asia, and the Pacific. Widowhood adds to the dilemma of older women. In Fiji, 14% of males and 52% of females are widowed. In Malaysia, 13% of males and 61% of females are widowed. This female domination of widowhood is common throughout most developing countries. Widowed women can be a burden to struggling young families due to their lower levels of education, poor prospects for employment, and more frequent health problems.

Elderly women appear as beggars on city streets in Guatemala, Colombia, Russia, China, Korea, and other countries. Women who are not able to contribute to the household are turned out into the streets or leave the household themselves so their children may have a larger share of the food or assets (Tout 1994). Widowhood increases social isolation for both men and women and loneliness is a major problem. Widowed persons are at greater risk for physical and mental health problems and financial instability.

Divorce acutely affects the lives of older men and women. Millions of young children live in single-parent families. Divorce changes the nature of the grandparent-grandchild relationship and changes the balance of resources in the extended family. Modern society's trend toward late-life divorces has negatively affected older women financially and socially and contributes to their mental and physical risks.

Employment and Retirement

The Department of Labor reports that 79.5% of men between the ages of 55 and 59 years and 54.8% of men aged 60 to 64 years are in the labor force. By age 65, only 16.6% are in the labor force. The number of older women in the work force is declining. More than 50% of all women aged 55 to 59 years are working, but only 8.4% of women older than 65 are employed. At age 60 to 64 years, 38% of black women, 36% of white women, and 34% of Hispanic women are employed.

Of the 2.9 million older adults working in 1990, less than half were on full-time schedules (U.S. Bureau of the Census 1996). Part-time employment is common among older persons. Older adults with pensions are less likely to continue working than are older adults who have Social Security income.

Discrimination against older employees is widespread in retirement programs or early retirement packages. Employers encourage early retirement in the United States by offering retirement incentive programs. Large corporations offer employees (usually at about age 50) lump-sum payments equal to six months' pay or even one year's salary if a person opts for early retirement.

Federal policy is discouraging early retirement to retain older workers in the labor force. In 2022, the retirement age will change from 65 to 67 years (Wacker, Roberto, and Piper 1998). Mandatory retirement age was prohibited by the 1986 amendments to the Age Discrimination in Employment Act of 1967. The United States Congress changed the Old Age and Survivor Insurance earnings test and, consequently, there are no longer earning limits for Social Security beneficiaries. Older-worker programs are discussed in another chapter. For information on Internet sites on this topic see Wacker, Roberto, and Piper's book: *Community Resources for Older Adults: Programs and Services in the Era of Change* (1998).

Sexuality

Sexuality refers to more than the biological functions of sexual inter-course and orgasm. Sexuality includes social and psychological issues of self-identity, expression of affection, intimacy, and satisfaction in rela-tionships. Positive or negative attitudes about sex and love in old age affect an older person's sexuality (Hooyman and Kiyak 1996). Illness, attitudes, and psychosocial factors may affect sexual activity. Ageism is responsible for society's negative attitudes toward sexuality in old age. Sexual attractiveness is equated with youth and physical appearance. While the physiological changes of aging usually do not affect sexual functioning, societal attitudes toward sexual expression in old age can have negative effects on the physical and mental well-being of older persons.

Studies of sexual activity generally use frequency of sexual inter-course as a measure of sexual activity. Using these measures, 25% of men were found to be impotent by age 70. Women reach a plateau of sexual activity in their sixties. The emphasis on frequency of sexual intercourse disregards the meaningfulness of the sexual activity. Although older adults may have sexual intercourse less often than do younger persons, the experience may be more meaningful.

Studies report that older persons are less interested in sex (sexual intercourse). Yet, studies that control for a cohort effect find stability in sexual activity throughout the life cycle. Conclusions are that persons who are sexually active in adulthood tend to be sexually active in mid-dle age and into old age. In 1981, Masters and Johnson found age–related physiological changes in both men and women, yet the capac-ity for sexual activity does not disappear (Hooyman and Kiyak 1996). Sexual activity remains stable throughout adulthood and may be more enjoyable in later life.

Age-related physiological changes that may affect sexual activity include postmenopausal changes (hot flashes, genital atrophy), urinary tract changes, and bone changes. Estrogen loss leads to genital atrophy, which is a reduction in the elasticity and lubrication of the vagina. The amount of lubricants secreted during sexual arousal diminishes and vaginal lubrication may take longer. While some discomfort may occur due to these changes, the use of lubricants such as vaginal jellies and creams minimizes the discomfort. Corbett and Gambrelin (1987) found that regular sexual activity, including masturbation, maintains vaginal lubricating ability and vaginal muscle tone and reduces discomfort during intercourse (Hooyman and Kiyak 1996). No impediment exists for women for full sexual activity throughout their lives. Women experience a slight decline in their capacity for sexual pleasure throughout their lives.

Men experience age-related physiological changes such as increase in length in the pre-orgasmic plateau phase, or excitement stage, and a slower response to direct stimulation. An erection may take longer to achieve and may require direct stimulation. Data reported by Theinhaus in 1988 stated that an 18-year-old male achieves a full erection on average in three seconds, at age 45 on average in eighteen to twenty seconds, and a 75-year-old man requires five minutes or more. The length of time between orgasm and subsequent erections is longer with greater age because of erective changes but these changes do not affect sexual fulfillment (Hooyman and Kiyak 1996, 249).

Impotence is unrelated to changes in sexual experience, but it is the chief cause for older men discontinuing sexual activity. Impotence may be psychological in nature or related to physical problems and use of medications. Age-related physiological changes in men and women do not interfere with sexual activity (Hooyman and Kiyak 1996).

Chronic illnesses can affect sexual functioning (i.e., heart disease, stroke, prostate disease, diabetes, and arthritis). Heart disease or heart attack may cause older adults to cease sexual activity and fear that sexual activity is life threatening. One of three men older than 65 years suffers from prostate problems. When prostate problems are treated by surgery, semen is no longer ejaculated through the penis, but is pushed back into the bladder and discharged through the urine. After healing, normal sexual functioning may return in some men. However, after radical prostatectomy is performed and nerves are cut, irreversible impotence occurs. Alternative treatments, such as radioactive pellet implantation, may be used.

Diabetics, particularly lifelong diabetics, may be impotent. Impotence in diabetics occurs because diabetes interferes with the circulatory mechanisms that supply blood flow to the penis for erection. For late-onset diabetics, impotence may be the first noted symptom; however, when diabetes is under control sexual activity can return to its previous state. Sexual functioning in women diabetics seems to be unimpaired.

Arthritis causes sexual activity to be painful and the pain-control medications may interfere with sexual desire and performance. Drugs and alcohol interfere with sexual desire and sexual functioning. Psychotropic drugs used to treat depression can impair erectile functioning. Hypertensive medications may affect sexual functioning. Gay and lesbian sexual issues in late life are discussed in another chapter in this book. The field of sexuality includes dating, remarriage, or friendships in late life.

Living Arrangements

In United States and in other countries, living environments can have a positive or negative impact upon the quality of life of older persons. The majority of older adults in the United States own the places in which they live. About 76% live in single-family dwellings, 13% live in multi-unit dwellings, 13% in semi-detached houses, and 5% in mobile homes (Wacker, Roberto, and Piper 1998). Because the majority of Americans own their homes, they spend a higher percentage of their incomes on their homes and are sometimes "house rich" and "cash poor."

A program that helps older adults remain in their homes is the Home Equity Conversion Program. Through this program, the homeowner borrows a lump sum from a bank with no repayment of the principal or interest until the homeowner either sells the house or dies. The reverse-mortgage program provides the borrower with monthly advances or a line of credit that can be used as needed. Payment is not due until the end of the loan term. Home-repair programs provide assistance with repairs. Funding for housing is provided by block grants from the Title III monies of the Older Americans Act. Home sharing is an arrangement in which two or more unrelated people share a home or apartment. Home sharers can share expenses or chores and provide each other with companionship.

Federal housing programs provide public housing for low-income persons. Rural programs assist with repair loans. Senior housing sites can be age-segregated housing communities or age-integrated housing. Planned retirement communities, such as Leisure World in California and Sun City in Arizona, offer amenities such as educational classes, tennis and golf, swimming, and recreational programs. Retirement communities are developing in Japan, Australia, New Zealand, and Europe.

Religion and Spirituality

Religion strongly influences the lives of older adults. Prayer, spirituality, and religiosity (defined in the literature as participation in places of worship) are reported to influence health—both physical and mental—and to buffer coping with the losses associated with aging (Koenig 1997).

Sixty-five percent of Americans identify themselves as Protestant, 25% as Catholic, and 3% as Jewish. More than 50% of older persons attend religious services at least once a week, and attendance at services tends to be positively related to well-being (Moody 1994). Koenig states, "Despite opinions to the contrary the vast majority of Americans still believe in God or some higher power" (1997, 33). In 1994, a Gallup poll reported that 94% of young Americans (18 to 29) believe in God while 97% of older Americans (age 50 and older) believe in God (Koenig 1997). As Table 5.1 illustrates, belief in God is worldwide.

A 1995 Gallup poll found that 58% of all Americans stated that religion was *very important* in their lives, while 73% of those older than 65 years stated that religion was *important* in their lives. In 1978, 52% of all Americans said that religion was *very important* in their lives, suggesting little change over the years. Religion's importance to Americans

Table 5.1 Belief in God Worldwide

Region	Percentage Who Believe in God
South America	95%
Australia	80%
Africa	96%
Europe	78%
Canada	89%

Source: Koenig, 1997

has not decreased since 1939. Most Americans are Protestant, with the largest groups being Baptist (22%), Methodist (9%), Lutheran (7%), Presbyterian (4%), Episcopal (2%), Pentecostal/Assembly of God (2%), nondenominational (6%), and other (7%).

Congregations are aging. More than 50% of members of mainline Protestant denominations are older than 60 years. Religious affiliation has remained stable since 1937, when 73% of Americans said they were members of churches or synagogues, while in 1994 more than 70% said they were religiously affiliated. Ninety percent of Americans pray (Koenig 1997).

Religion is more important than sports to Americans. In 1992, Americans spent $4 billion on sporting events while they donated $57 billion to religious causes. In 1993, 388 million people attended sporting events including tennis, soccer, and auto and dog racing, while at the same time attendance at local churches and synagogues was 5 billion (Koenig 1997).

A growing body of literature discusses the importance of spirituality in the lives of older adults. Spirituality is defined as a belief in a higher being. Ellor, Netting, and Thibault argue, "Religion and spirituality have the potential to act as coping mechanisms, sources of growth and self-transcendence, or sources of pathology for clients and practitioners alike" (1999, 114). In 1957, a seminal study reported frequent church attenders as being more open to the use of professional help for psychological problems. The church has a long history of support and aid in social problems (Taylor 1993; Tobin, Ellor, and Anderson-Ray 1986). Religiousness, whether described as institutional or personal, is correlated positively with better morale, stronger coping skills, and better physical and mental health. Depression and alcohol abuse are less prevalent in religious older adults. Hypertension, anxiety, and cardiac problems are influenced by religious behaviors (Krause 1991; Markides et al. 1987). Religious older persons are less depressed and have better mental health than do non-religious older persons (Koenig, George, and Siegler 1988). Studies report a strong link between religiosity and life satisfaction (Koenig, George, and Siegler 1988). Koenig and colleagues document the positive association between religion and health, particularly mental health, in studies from Duke University (Koenig 1995).

Controversy exists regarding the measurement and conceptualization of the concepts of religion, religiosity, and spirituality. Johnson (1995) explains differences between the subjective and the behavioral dimension of religion. The subjective dimension refers to intrinsic factors such as religious commitment and how vital religion is to the person. The behavioral dimension or extrinsic factors refer to attendance or involvement in church activities. Tirrito and Spencer-Amado (2000) studied the functional role of the church in the lives of older adults.

Leisure Activities

Longer life expectancies and earlier retirement allow more time and opportunity for leisure activities for older persons. Participation in leisure activities offers several benefits to older persons. It replaces a work role, increases preretirement interests, maintains a positive self-concept, and enhances mental health (Wacker, Roberto, and Piper 1998). Leisure activities provide companionship and informal social-support networks. Leisure activities include: passive activities—television, hobbies, and crafts; social activities—visiting with friends and participation in social organizations; and physical activities—swimming and walking. Higher levels of participation in hobbies, crafts, social organizations, and visiting with friends are significantly related to higher levels of psychological well-being (Wacker, Roberto, and Piper 1998).

Americans are retired more years than ever before. Early retirement has changed the focus of retirement from a time of role loss to the pursuit of personal fulfillment. Americans are retiring early and pursing travel, education, and personal achievements. Older adults try out new leisure activities such as skydiving, rafting, scuba diving, hot air ballooning, and mountain climbing. Older persons are pursuing second and third careers in colleges and universities. Law school at age 60, medical school at age 50, and college degrees at age 70 are no longer rare.

Technological communication and computers are important leisure and educational pursuits for seniors, and in Europe and the United States older adults are a large market for computer technology businesses. The Eurobarometer Survey of 1997, a survey conducted by the Brussels-based European Commission to gauge the European

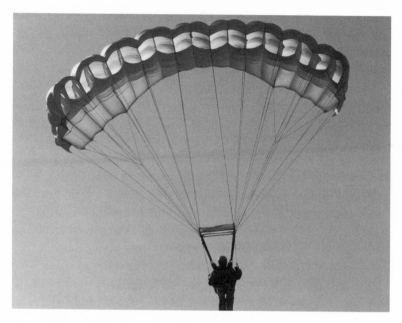

Older adults are trying more active forms of leisure such as skydiving.

community's views on public access to the Internet, found that in Germany 11.4% of older adults (older than 55 years) use computers; in France, 7.5% use computers; 11% in the United Kingdom; and 5% in the Netherlands. In the United States, 30% of people older than 50 years own and use a personal computer. A study done by Microsoft and the American Society on Aging cited in *Aging Today Newsletter* (1999) at http://www. asaging.org, found that ownership rates drop with age. Only 16% of those ages 70–79 years own and use computers. According to a SeniorNet study in 1998, 16.5% of the total online population is older than 50 years (Gilligan 1999).

Summary

Biological research explores the body's aging process, and psychological research studies behaviors and lifestyles. Social gerontologists examine the impact of the social environment. In this chapter, attention was given to the biopsychosocial aspects of aging because the quality of life of older persons is powerfully influenced by health, psychological status, spirituality, and the social environment. Biology and lifestyles determine health status. Psychological status is influenced by health status as well as the social environment and spirituality. The interaction of biology, psychology, and social environment is obvious and knowledge of older persons must be examined from a biopsychosocial perspective.

References

Belsky, Janet. 1990. *The psychology of aging: Theory, research, and interventions.* 2nd ed. Pacific Grove, Calif.: Brooks/Cole Publishing.

Birren, J. E., and B. A. Birren. 1990. The concepts, models and history of the psychology of aging. In *Handbook of the psychology of aging,* edited by J. E. Birren and K. W. Schaie. 3rd ed. San Diego, Calif.: Academic Press.

Birren, J. E., and J. J. F. Schoots. 1996. History, concepts, and theory in the psychology of aging. In *Handbook of the psychology of aging,* edited by J. E. Birren and K. W. Schaie. 4th ed. San Diego, Calif.: Academic Press.

Dychtwald, K. 1995. *Middlescence and beyond.* Videotape. Emeryville, Calif: Age Wave.

Ellor, James W., Ellen F. Netting, and Jane M. Thibault. 1999. *Religious and spiritual aspects of human service practice.* Columbia: Univ. of South Carolina Press.

France, Anne-Claire. 1990. Psychology of aging: Stability and change in intelligence and personality. In *Gerontology: Perspectives and issues,* edited by Kenneth Ferraro. New York: Springer Publishing.

Geralnik, David, ed. 1974. *Webster's new world dictionary.* 2nd ed. New York: Williams Collins and World Publishing.

Gilligan, Rosemarie. 1999. Getting elders wired: Progress report on Europe and the U.S. *Aging Today* 20 (6): 13.

Hooyman, N., and H. A. Kiyak. 1996. *Social gerontology: A multidisciplinary perspective.* 4th ed. Boston: Allyn and Bacon.

Johnson, T. 1995. The significance of religion for aging well. *American Behavioral Scientist* 39 (2): 186–208.

Kimmel, Douglas C. 1990. *Adulthood and aging.* New York: John Wiley and Sons.

Koenig, H. 1997. *Is religion good for your health? The effects of religion on physical and mental health.* New York: Haworth Press.

Koenig, H. G., L. George, and I. C. Siegler. 1988. The use of religion and other emotion-regulating coping strategies among older adults. *Gerontologist* 28: 303–10.

Krause, N. 1991. Stress, religiosity, and abstinence from alcohol. *Psychology and Aging* 6: 134–44.

Levinson, G. 1978. *The seasons of a man's life.* New York: Knopf.

Markides, K. S., J. S. Levin, and L. R. Ray. 1987. Religion, aging, and life satisfaction: An eight-year, three-wave longitudinal study. *Gerontologist* 27: 660–65.

Moody, Harry R. 1994. *Aging: Concepts and controversies.* Thousand Oaks, Calif.: Pine Forge Press.

National Institute of Health, National Institute on Aging. 1993. *In search of the secrets of aging.* Bethesda, Md.: Public Information Office. On-line: http://www.nih.gov/health/chip/nia/aging/quest.html#life.

Neugarten, B., R. Havighurst, and S. Tobin. 1968. Personality and patterns of aging. In *Middle age and aging,* edited by Bernice Neugarten. Chicago: Univ. of Chicago Press.

Peck, Robert. 1968. Psychological developments in the second half of life. In *Middle age and aging,* edited by Bernice Neugarten. Chicago: Univ. of Chicago Press.

Pruncho, Rachel. 1999. Raising grandchildren: The experiences of black and white grandmothers. *Gerontologist* 39 (2): 202–21.

Salthouse, T. A. 1990. Speed of behavior and the implications for cognition. In *Handbook of the psychology of aging.* 3rd ed. Edited by J. E. Birren and K. W. Schaie. San Diego, Calif.: Academic Press.

Schaie, K. W. 1996. Intellectual development in adulthood. In *Handbook of the psychology of aging.* 4th ed. Edited by J. E. Birren and K. W. Schaie. San Diego, Calif.: Academic Press.

Schneider, E. L., and J. W. Rowe, eds. 1996. *Handbook of the biology of aging.* 4th ed. San Diego, Calif.: Academic Press.

Taylor, Robert. 1993. Religion and religious observances. In *Aging in black America,* edited by J. S. Jackson, L. M. Chatters, and R. J. Taylor. Newberry Park, Calif.: Sage Publications.

Tirrito, T., and J. Spencer-Amado. 2000. Older adults' willingness to use social services in places of worship. *Journal of Religious Gerontology* 11 (2): 29–43.

Tobin, S, M. Ellen, J. Ellor, and S. Anderson-Ray. 1986. *Enabling the elderly: Religious institutions within the community service system.* Albany: State Univ. of New York Press.

Tout, Ken. 1994. Grandparents as parents in developing countries. *Aging International* 21 (1) (Mar.): 19–24.

U.S. Bureau of the Census. 1996. *Current Population Reports, Special Studies. P23–190, 65+ in the United States.* Washington, D.C.: GPO.

Wacker, Robbyn R., Kenneth Roberto, and Linda E. Piper. 1998. *Community resources for older adults: Programs and services in the era of change.* Thousand Oaks, Calif.: Pine Forge Press.

CHAPTER SIX

Sociological Theories of Aging

Sociological theories of aging are influenced by theories in sociology. Sociology emerged with the works of Emile Durkheim, Max Weber, and Karl Marx. Matcha defines sociological theories as "a set of assumptions concerning society and social phenomena in reference to their separate societal reality" or, more broadly, "an explanation system of social phenomena" (1996, 47). While sociological theories explain social phenomena, sociological theories of aging attempt to explain social phenomena and their relationship to the aging individual.

One important sociological theory is *structural functionalism,* often referred to as functionalism. The major concept in this theory is "function," which refers to the consequences of an "action." The concept of "structure" refers to the organizational level or societal level. Matcha (1996, 48) describes functionalism in the following way:

- ❖ Social systems are composed of interconnected parts.
- ❖ Social systems confront external and internal problems of survival.
- ❖ Such problems of survival can be visualized as the "needs" or "requisites" of the system.
- ❖ Social systems and their constituent parts can only be understood by assessing how a part contributes to meeting the needs or requisites of the systemic whole.

Matcha (1996) writes that functionalist theorists propose that differences based on age are legitimate aspects of the social order. Society creates structures because they are functional for the society. Retirement and pensions are functional systems created because they are functional for society. Retirement provides job opportunities for younger persons to enter the workforce, and pensions offer income security for retirees.

In modern societies retirement includes income security. The function of retirement is not appropriate for all members of society. Older adults who are poor are unable to retire and often work as long as possible. Retirement does not serve a positive function for older adults who wish to work and are forced to retire. Because mandatory retirement is illegal in the United States, alternative methods are used to force retirement such as the "early out." In this option, incentives are given to older workers to leave the workforce while younger workers are hired who are paid less money.

European older adults retire earlier and are pensioners by age 60 years. In the United States, there is a trend toward early retirement. The function of retirement has changed in modern society.

Symbolic interactionism, another important sociological theory, explains the use of symbols for communication. A symbol is anything—such as a flag, baptism, wedding, bar mitzvah, or funeral—that gives meaning to a concept. Matcha (1996) describes basic assumptions of symbolic interactionism:

- Human beings act toward things on the basis of the meanings the things have for them.
- These meanings are the products of social interaction in human society.
- These meanings are modified and handled through an interpretative process used by each individual in dealing with the signs each encounters.

Older adults act toward aging on the basis of meanings society attaches to old age. The negativism of aging is self-fulfilling. In a society that supports education primarily for young people, older adults learn that older persons are too old to learn a new task, a new language, or a new activity. When societal attitudes depict primarily young people as being beautiful and sexy, older adults learn negative self-images regarding attractiveness and sexuality.

In the so-called "celebration" of birthdays for older persons, age 50 is described as "over the hill," sexless, an age at which to plan retirement, the beginning of physical decline, etc. In some cultures, birthdays in the later years are times of celebration. In Korea, age 60 is a time of celebration with several days of festivities. There is a story of a group of elders in the mountains of Tibet who reported a majority of their population to be older than 100 years old. Upon scientific investigation, it was found that in this culture age was greatly exaggerated to enhance status.

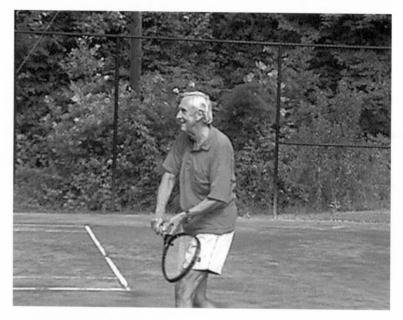

Tennis player confirms the activity theory.

Sociological and anthropological theories influenced theories of aging—such as disengagement theory, activity theory, exchange theory, and continuity theory. Other gerontological theories, the modernization theory, the feminist approach, and the political economy perspective, are also useful in understanding attitudes and roles of older persons in various societies. Figures on pages 123 and 124 illustrate the interaction of sociological theories and gerontological theories and the linkages of the theories of disengagement, activity, and exchange to structural functionalism and symbolic interactionism.

Disengagement Theory

Disengagement theory is an eminent gerontological theory. From this theoretical perspective, the structural functionalist describes disengagement as being functional for both society and the individual. It is deemed necessary for individuals to withdraw from society to allow younger persons to participate in the society. Retirement serves an important function for society by providing job opportunities for young persons. In 1960, the disengagement theory was described in an article by Cummings, Dean, Newell, and McCaffery. The theory was popularized by Cummings and Henry in 1961 in their work, *Growing Old*. The disengagement theory is based on the Kansas City study of 275 middle-aged and older-aged persons. A linear relationship between age and disengagement was reported; for example, as a person ages disengagement becomes greater. *Disengagement* is removal or withdrawal from previous activities. Disengagement ends with the death of the person.

The process of disengagement is mutual and universal; that is, disengagement occurs across cultures, and the process is inevitable and functional for society. One of the earliest attempts to explain old age in modern society is the disengagement theory (Moody 1994). The disengagement theory is described as a natural tendency to give up certain functions and responsibilities. For example, society requires a police officer to retire at an earlier age than the usual 65 years because physical strength is believed to diminish with age. Sports figures must leave professional careers while still in their twenties or thirties. From the perspective of disengagement theory, retirement is the process of

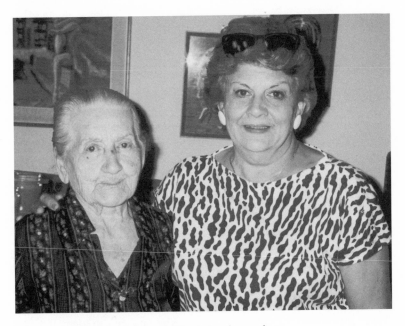

Emotional support is a large part of social exchange theory.

mutual withdrawal between the individual and society and is beneficial for both the individual and society. However, there is little empirical evidence that older persons want to disengage from society.

Neugarten, Havighurst, and Tobin (1968) found that, in middle age, the individual becomes more involved in an inner psychological world, which they termed "interiority." Concern with outward achievement lessens as interest in self-development or spirituality becomes more prominent. The ability to detach from certain functions and responsibilities demonstrates flexibility in coping with the changes of advancing years. From this perspective, disengagement is a positive coping mechanism. As one disengages from societal responsibilities, there is concern with generativity. *Generativity* is leaving a mark on the world or leaving something of one's self to the world.

From the symbolic interactionist perspective, society disengages the older adult from the work force by setting age 65 as pension-eligible age. Another symbol forcing the older person to retire is the attitude that older persons lose physical capability and should leave physically demanding jobs such as flying airplanes, law enforcement, and sports.

Activity Theory

Activity theory became popular in the United States in 1949. It was proposed by Cavan, Burgess, Havinghurst, and Goldhamer, and again in 1953 by Havinghurst and Albrect. It became widely known after the emergence of the disengagement theory. This perspective, which is counter to the disengagement theory, argues that involvement with society is essential for life satisfaction. Proponents believe that individuals age successfully if they maintain their prior activity levels (Matcha 1996). The activity theory connected well to American values of hard work, staying active, and maintaining independence. Activity brings happiness in old age, and persons who are not active will not be happy.

In the 1970s, proponents of the activity theory influenced programs and policies and insisted that activity was necessary for a satisfying old age. Senior centers, retirement communities, senior employment programs, and volunteering would bring happiness to older persons. Work and activity are necessary to avoid an unhappy old age, and retirement is withdrawal from the world and leads to stagnation and early death. Moody writes, "The ideal of active aging seems in many respects

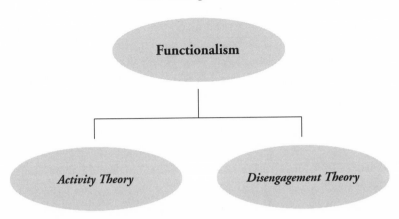

Sociological Theories and Aging Theories

a prolongation of middle age rather than something special or distinctive about the last stage of life" (1994, 76). Although the activity theory influenced programs and added to the quality of life for older adults, it also contributed to the misperception that older people must be busy to be happy.

Based on this perspective, legislation required nursing homes to employ recreation workers and develop activity programs to keep residents involved and busy. Residents who cannot or do not participate in recreational programs are seen as disadvantaged. Although this theoretical perspective has been challenged by researchers, it lingers in social attitudes. Senior centers, adult day-care centers, assisted-living centers, and residential-care centers advocate that keeping busy is the key to happiness in old age.

Continuity Theory

"Continuity theory addresses aging as an evolutionary, dynamic process in which change is inevitable and necessary" (Matcha 1996, 58). According to this theory, individuals maintain consistent patterns of activity throughout their lifetimes. Continuity requires social relationships and a societal environment that supports lifetime experiences.

Continuity theory argues that older individuals must maintain earlier life activities or experiences for stability. For example, the individual who enjoys quiet walks in the park, reading, and small group activities will enjoy the same or similar activities in old age. If the young person is involved in church activities, the older person will most likely remain involved in the church. The young person who is a sports enthusiast will most likely remain one. The musician, artist, and traveler will most likely continue to enjoy these activities in old age.

However, if the social or physical environment prohibits that activity, stress will result. For example, when relocation changes the social environment, stress results because activities are no longer possible (Matcha 1996). Relocation to a nursing home, to a child's home, or to the hospital are stressful experiences. Relocation to a retirement community can be a stressful or a positive experience. The support of the environment (society) is necessary for the individual to maintain continuity throughout the life cycle and, thus, maintain stability (Kart 1997).

While continuity in activities is the optimum choice, social, psychological, or physical factors can be barriers for continuity. Tomorrow's healthier, more active older adults will prefer to continue their same activities for a much longer time, but they will also expect support from the environment.

Social Exchange Theory

Symbolic interactionism influences the application of the social exchange theory to aging. A mutual exchange exists between older persons and younger persons in the form of support (emotional, financial, and instrumental). The exchange theory may not be appropriate for

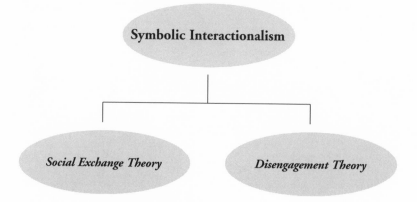

Sociological Theories and Aging Theories

aging if the old have few resources to contribute to the young (Marshall 1996). When older persons are unable to provide an exchange of services, the result is marginalization of older persons and a loss of respect for themselves and from others (Albert and Cattell 1994).

In societies in which late-life dependency is not a negative state but is expected and desired, such as in Asian countries, the exchange of love for assistance is a balanced exchange. In African countries, childless women raise unrelated kin, assuming there will be an exchange of caregiving in later life.

Mutual support is provided by the young and the old. A 1979 cross-national study by Shanas found that older adults in the United States, England, and Denmark are not abandoned by their families (Moody 1994). Older adults provide a great deal of support to younger family members in the form of money and services (Riley and Foner 1968). The amount of support given or received has little effect on the feelings of obligation to others (Kart 1997). For centuries western and eastern societies exchanged help between generations in the form of accumulated wealth and inheritance as a means of transfer of goods. Older persons, usually fathers, pass their wealth to children to support their own families from the inheritance. In most cultures, the mantle is passed from the old to the young to manage societies.

Inheritance in the form of passing of land has lessened, but in New Zealand, family inheritance supports the next generation of the family. Currently in New Zealand's economy, the young have little savings and the older person, who previously passed his farm to his son, now must sell the land. The son, who would have raised his family with the inheritance of the land, now struggles to support his own family. Although financial exchange from the older to the younger members seems to be lessening, there is evidence that emotional and social support between the young and the old remains stable (St. John 1993).

Social exchange occurs in friendships. Equal exchange is not important in best-friend relationships, but concern for equality is important in secondary-acquaintance relationships (Albert and Cattell 1994). The social exchange theory in modern societies takes the form of reciprocal care and services. Benefits to older persons and from older persons to younger persons are the basis for intergenerational equity. Intergenerational programs, with the old and young helping each other, will have a significant effect on relationships between the old and the young. The healthier, better educated, older baby boomer has the ability to provide assistance to younger members of societies.

Other Theoretical Approaches

Other theoretical approaches will be discussed briefly. The *feminist approach* reflects a commitment to use a certain perspective and examines the neglect of attention to gender in work, family, and social stratification (Marshall 1996). Arber and Ginn in *Gender and Later Life* focus on inequalities and differences in the way aging affects men and women and describe aging as being a "gendered process" (1991, 2).

The feminization of poverty describes older women as being more at risk for poverty. *Double jeopardy* is a term that refers to a woman who is old and female as being at risk in society. The older woman is disadvantaged and at risk for poverty in developed and developing countries. Older women are economically disadvantaged. Older poor women are dependent upon family members for support. In India, Japan, and China, the son and daughter-in-law provide support and care for the older woman. One possible exchange of services is providing child care in exchange for financial support. In societies where females are devalued, the older woman is at great risk for abandonment and neglect. In Russia, a country currently struggling with its political process and economy, older women are not uncommonly homeless and street beggars. In difficult economic times, children cannot support their dependent parents so that older persons are at greater risk.

Modernization theory portrays the aging individual as being negatively impacted by modern society—being roleless and devalued. This theory is popular in developing countries where changes in the social structure influence changes in the family structure. For example, in Korea the responsibilities of modern families are changing the contributory role of the older person. Day-care centers provide care for children so that older family members are not needed to care for young children.

As societies move from agricultural societies to industrialized societies, attitudes toward older persons become more negative (Baiyewu et al. 1997). Chinese people living in Taiwan had a more positive attitude toward elders than did poeple in a Chinese group living in the United States (Baiyewu et al. 1997). The attitudes of Samoans living in

Honolulu and those living in American Samoa and rural Western Samoa differed, and Samoans living in Honolulu and American Samoa had more negative attitudes toward their elders. India and Nigeria report a positive attitude toward elders. In Nigeria elders maintain a role in the major religious ceremonies of the society, such as marriages and naming ceremonies of newborn babies.

A study of the aged in rural Kenya reports that older persons without children suffer from lack of help. The tradition of respecting the old is changing in the People's Republic of China and Hong Kong. A study by Chow, which examined the perception of old age by both aged and young respondents, found the status and roles of the elders among the Chinese are changing. The practice of filial piety or *Xaio* has, for thousands of years, been described as respecting the old. While the practice is still upheld among Chinese all over the world, there is evidence that older people are finding themselves less revered when their experiences become less valuable (Chow 1999).

Modernization theory proposes that the decreased value of the older person is a by-product of technological change and decreasing need for the skills of older persons (Cavanaugh 1996). In agricultural societies, old age provides valuable experiences. In modern technological societies, the learning experiences of older persons are replaced by formal educational systems. The modernization of societies may be responsible for the loss of prestige and power of older adults in society (Cavanaugh 1996). The least-modernized societies (Iraq, El Salvador, and the Philippines) show the greatest degree of equality in employment between young and old. Highly modernized societies (Norway, the Netherlands) show a decline in equality between old and young and a lower economic status for older persons. Societies in the upper levels of development show an improvement in the status of older persons (Albert and Cattell 1994).

The *political economy perspective* directs attention to the treatment of older people in society and the experience of old age and its relationship to the economy of the country. Proponents argue that society's treatment of the aged is related to the economy; the conditions of the labor market; and the class, race, sex, and age divisions in a society. Estes (1991, 31) explains the structure of the political economy of aging:

1. Social structure shapes how older adults are perceived and how they perceive themselves.

2. Labels applied to the elderly shape the experience of old age and influence policy decisions for the elderly.

3. Social policy reflects the dominant ideology and belief systems that enforce the structure of advantage and disadvantage in the larger economic, political, and social order.

From this perspective, we look beyond the elderly as a social problem to the causes and conditions of societal problems that depict aging as a social problem. When the economy demands that the young work in urban areas, the aged are left behind in an environment that lacks support from productive workers. Rural areas are unable to support older adults without productive workers. The impact on social behaviors of changes in control of resources is evident in a report from American Samoa, where a decline in elder authority transformed the entire social economy. In the past, common people gave all of their fish to the chief and he distributed the fish among the people in an entrepreneurial system that revolved around wage labor and family consumption. The fisherman no longer gives his fish to the chief; rather, he manages his own catch. The ability of the older person to control resources and to maintain prestige in the community is eliminated, and the older person's status is diminished at the same time that he is no longer able to support himself.

In Singapore, a highly modern society, the young are financially responsible for the care of parents. In a society where the young are educated and capable of financial independence or the wealth of the society is based on new technology and the aged no longer control the resources, there is economic inequality. A substantial proportion of older persons in the United States, particularly women, are in dire circumstances (Albert and Cattell 1994). The political economy perspective attempts to explain attitudes and behaviors toward older persons by examining the political economy of the society.

Summary

Sociological theories explain the nature of society and how people behave in a society. The interaction between sociological theories and theories of aging is evident in the disengagement theory, activity theory, life continuity theory, and social exchange theory. Theories of the past century explain attitudes toward older adults and the behaviors of young and old. The next century will bring new perspectives to explain attitudes and behaviors. Baby boomers will retire earlier, work part-time at new jobs, be more spiritual, pursue challenging leisure activities, be physically active and energetic, and have more added years to provide intergenerational support to the young.

Technology will change the lives of baby boomers, offering opportunities to learn new skills, to work at non-traditional jobs, and to interact with geographically distant families. Maintaining relationships and offering emotional assistance to family members may be easier because of telecommunications. Social exchanges with family and friends in various parts of the country or the world are possible. Grandparents can see and learn about their grandchildren, from America to France or Korea to Russia. Transfer of information through computers allows for worldwide exchange of ideas, advice, and gifts. A new world of technology is available for the next cohort of older persons—the baby boomers. In the next millennium, older adults, their children, and their grandchildren will have opportunities to share their ideas, cultures, histories, and current lives with their families through the use of computers, television, telephones, and new forms of communication technology yet to be developed. It promises to be an exciting future.

References

Albert, Steven M., and Maria G. Cattell. 1994. *Old age in global perspective: Cross cultural and cross national views.* New York. Macmillan.

Arber, S., and J. Ginn. 1991. *Gender and later life: Resources and constraints.* London: Sage Publications.

Baiyewu, O., A. F. Bella, J. D. Adeyemi, B. A. Ikuesan, E. A. Bamgboye, and R. O. Jegede. 1997. Attitudes toward aging among different groups in Nigeria. *International Journal of Aging and Human Development* 44 (4): 283–92.

Cavanaugh, John. C. 1996. *Adult development and aging.* 3rd ed. Pacific Grove, Calif.: Brooks/Cole Publishers.

Chow, Nelson. 1999. Diminishing filial piety and the changing role and status of elders in Hong Kong. *Hallym International Journal of Aging* 1 (1): 67–77.

Estes, C. L. 1991. The new political economy of aging: Introduction and critique. In *Critical perspectives on aging: The political and moral economy of growing old,* edited by M. Minkleer and C. L. Estes. Amityville, N.Y.: Baywood.

Kart, Cary S. 1997. *The realities of aging: An introduction to gerontology.* 5th ed. Boston: Allyn and Bacon.

Marshall, Victor. 1996. The state of theory in aging and the social sciences. In *Handbook of aging and the social sciences,* edited by R. H. Binstock and L. K. George. 4th ed. San Diego, Calif.: Academic Press.

Matcha, Duane. 1996. *The sociology of aging: A social problems perspective.* Boston: Allyn and Bacon.

Moody, Harry R. 1994. *Aging: Concepts and controversies.* Thousand Oaks, Calif.: Pine Forge Press.

Neugarten, B., R. Havighurst, and S. Tobin. 1968. Personality and patterns of aging. In *Middle age and aging,* edited by Bernice Neugarten. Chicago: Univ. of Chicago Press.

Riley, M., and A. Foner. 1968. *An inventory of research findings.* Vol. 1 of *Aging and Society.* New York: Russell Sage Foundation.

St. John, Susan. 1993. Income support for an aging society. In *New Zealand's aging society: The implications,* edited by Peggy Koopman-Boyden. Wellington, New Zealand: Daphne Brasell Associates Press.

CHAPTER SEVEN

Health and Diseases

The physical and mental health of older adults is of importance in the study of aging persons. Health is a major determinant of quality of life and longevity. The quality of life of older adults is seriously impacted by health problems. Heart disease is the leading cause of death in all industrialized countries. In the last decade, there was a decline in deaths from heart disease in some countries. Chronic diseases, which particularly affect women, are more common in an aging population.

Mental health problems affect quality of life. The most common problems for older persons are dementia, Alzheimer's disease, alcoholism, anxiety disorders, drug abuse, and depression. It is essential to have a comprehensive understanding of the incidence and prevalence of physical and mental illnesses that plague older adults.

Health of Older Adults

Health is defined by the World Health Organization (1947) as a state of complete physical, mental, and social well-being. This definition is widely used. Health implies an integration of body, mind, and spirit (Hooyman and Kiyak 1996). Health status refers to the presence or absence of disease and the degree of disability in an individual's level of functioning. A commonly used measure of functioning is the ADL, or Activities of Daily Living. The ADL measures a person's ability to manage personal care in five areas: eating, bathing, dressing, toileting, and mobility.

The costs of health care are rising as a result of the increasing numbers of older persons and their need for care. This trend is alarming around the world. In the United States, the Medicare costs for inpatient and outpatient care and long-term care costs (U.S. Bureau of the Census 1992) are issues for political debates. A considerable proportion of public-health dollars is spent on the care of the elderly in most developed countries. In the United States, 58% of public health dollars was spent on the elderly in 1987, up from 51% in 1977. In 1987, personal health-care expenditures averaged approximately $3,700 for persons ages 65 to 69 years, and approximately $9,200 for persons ages 85 years and older. Hospitalization accounts for most expenditures. In 1991, $60 billion was spent on nursing-home care in the United States (Koster and Prather 1998).

Health and disability status among the elderly improved worldwide between 1982 and 1995; consequently, poor health is not as prevalent as it was three decades ago, especially among the young-old. The National Institutes of Health and National Institute on Aging (1993) reported that 75% of non-institutionalized persons ages 65 to 74 years consider their health to be good, very good, or excellent compared to others their age. More than 66% of non-institutionalized persons older than 75 years also considered their health to be good, very good, or excellent. The percent of those persons who identify their health as good, very good, or excellent has risen over the past twenty years.

Healthy agers are persons who are free of physical-performance limitations, chronic conditions, limitations of activities of daily living, and who report their health as good, very good, or excellent. However, the

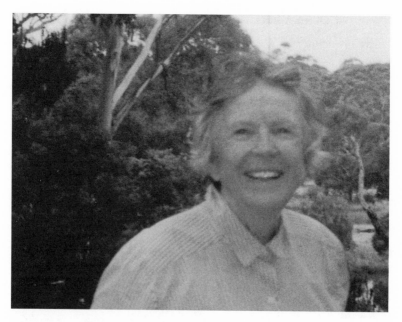

The founder of the School of Social Work of the University of Papua, New Guinea, continues to contribute to life by lecturing in Australian schools of social work.

need for personal assistance with everyday activities increases with age. Among persons ages 15 to 64 years, only 2% need assistance; at ages 65 to 69 the percent of those needing assistance rises to 9%, and it rises higher, to 50% for those persons ages 85 and older. Functional limitations are more prevalent among women than men. Elderly African American persons have higher rates of functional limitations than do elderly white persons. Yet in spite of these limitations older persons worldwide are enjoying better health and increased years to live (Koster and Prather 1998).

Common Acute and Chronic Diseases

In developed countries, the leading causes of mortality for older men and older women are diseases of the heart, cancer, cerebrovascular diseases, and chronic pulmonary obstructive diseases. The incidence of circulatory diseases (heart disease, stroke, and hypertension) increases with age. While incidence of these diseases declined in the last forty years, they remain the leading causes of death among older persons worldwide. For example, more than half of all deaths of older persons in Argentina, Bulgaria, and the United States are attributed to circulatory diseases (U.S. Bureau of the Census 1992).

Among adults ages 35 years and older, heart disease is the leading cause of death in developing countries. Deaths from cancer are next. In France, the United Kingdom, Belgium, Finland, and the Netherlands, there has been a decline of 10% to 20% in deaths from heart disease. In North America, death rates declined almost 50% from the 1960s. In Greece, Yugoslavia, and some Eastern European nations, mortality from heart disease increased 20% to 40%. In the United States, the leading cause of death is still heart disease, but among those ages 65 to 74 years, heart disease and cancer were equally prevalent causes of death. An analysis of heart disease by gender in twenty-six countries found that male rates had a variety of patterns; female rates decreased among persons ages 45 to 64 years (U.S. Bureau of the Census 1992).

Overall, deaths from cancer have risen 30% to 50% among men since 1950 while they have decreased approximately 10% for women. In the United States and Western Europe, stomach cancer has declined since the 1930s, a decline attributed to a reduction of salt in food, especially in preserved food. Lung cancer increased since the 1950s, initially among men and later among women. Increased rates of smoking in Asian and Eastern European countries contributed to increased rates of cancer in these regions. Male deaths appear to be falling, as in Finland and the United Kingdom, and they are stabilizing in other countries. While lung cancer rose among women, breast cancer remains the principal site of neoplasms among women. Mortality rates from breast cancer have increased in most countries since 1945. The rise is most evident in Southern and Eastern Europe, a fact consistent with the hypothesis that diets high in saturated fat are risk factors for breast cancer.

Epidemiological transition indicates a change in leading causes of death from infectious and acute diseases to chronic and degenerative diseases (U.S. Bureau of the Census 1992). The leading causes of death in South Korea from 1966 to 1991 are listed in table 7.1. Widespread use of antibiotics is responsible for the change in causes of death from pneumonia and bronchitis to cancer and heart disease.

Chronic diseases of the aged include arthritis, osteoporosis, kidney diseases, hypertension, diabetes, and Alzheimer's disease. These diseases contribute to long-term health problems and dependency. Doctors are able to save the lives of people who, decades ago, would have died from heart disease; however, these individuals live out their lives with other

Table 7.1 Leading Causes of Death in South Korea

1966	**1981**	**1991**
Pneumonia	Malignant Neoplasms	Malignant Neoplasms
Tuberculosis	Hypertension	Cerebrovascular
Cerebrovascular	Cerebrovascular	Senile Disease
Other Infections	Non-Traffic Accidents	Pulmonary
Malignant Neoplasms	Senile Disease	Non-Traffic Accidents
All Accidents	Chronic Liver Disease	Traffic Accidents
Bronchitis	Traffic Accidents	Hypertension
Meningitis	Tuberculosis	Chronic Liver Disease
Hypertension	Suicide	Other Circulatory Diseases

Source: Choe, 1989

chronic illnesses. The percentage of persons ages 65 and older who visit a physician increased in the past several decades (U.S. Bureau of the Census 1992). Health problems associated with the three major causes of death (heart disease, malignant neoplasms, and cerebrovascular diseases) include smoking, alcohol abuse, and poor diet.

Elderly African American men are twice as likely to smoke as are white men. More than half of elderly men and one-third of elderly women use alcohol. Heavy drinkers incur higher mortality risks from liver cirrhosis, cancers, hypertension, and diabetes.

Poor diet is a contributor to heart disease. In the United States, 68% of men and 71% of women older than 65 years are classified as overweight. Higher proportions of men and women between ages 35 and 64 years are overweight than in previous years.

As chronological age increases, multiple chronic illnesses increase. Women are more likely to have two or more common chronic conditions (referred to as co-morbidity) than men. Studies indicate that, among those 80 years and older, 70% of women and 53% of men have two or more common chronic conditions (U.S. Bureau of the Census 1992). Most changes—wrinkling of the skin, graying of the hair, some sensory and/or hearing changes, changes in muscle tone—are attributed to normal aging rather than to pathological conditions.

Mental Health and Aging

Mental health problems of the older population are influenced by social structures such as family, community and institutional care, ethnic and cultural differences, socioeconomic status, and physical problems. The *Handbook of Mental Health and Aging* (Birren, Sloane, and Cohen 1992) is recommended for a review of mood disorders, personality disorders, schizophrenia, and psychotic states. The most prevalent mental health problems in older persons are Alzheimer's disease or related dementia, depression, anxiety disorders, drug abuse, and alcoholism.

Dementia

Dementia is a syndrome or a group of symptoms that affect cognitive functioning. Dementia may be caused by numerous disorders. The most significant feature of dementia is impairment in short- and long-term memory.

Dementia is diagnosed when at least four of the following conditions are present:

❖ Impairment in abstract thinking.
❖ Impaired judgment.
❖ Personality change.
❖ Disturbances of cortical functions such as aphasia, apraxia, agnosia, and constructional difficulty.
❖ Impairment in short- and long-term memory.
(Raskind and Peskind 1992)

In order for dementia to be diagnosed, these disturbances must be significant and must interfere with work, social activities, and relationships with others. There must be evidence of organic etiology or the presence of a psychiatric illness such as major depression. Dementia can be reversible when it is caused by normal pressure hydrocephalus, brain tumors, depression, medication, vitamin deficiency, hypothyroidism, or toxic substances (National Institute on Aging and National Institutes of Health 1996). Dementia is easily misdiagnosed and its symptoms attributed to causes other than pathology.

Alzheimer's Disease

Worldwide, the number of persons with Alzheimer's disease (AD) is estimated to be 12 million, and 22 million are expected to have Alzheimer's disease by 2025. In the United States, an estimated 4 million people have Alzheimer's disease (National Institute on Aging and National Institutes of Health 1996). An estimated 19 million persons in the United States say they have a family member with Alzheimer's disease, and 37 million say they know someone who has the disease (Alzheimer's Association 2000). Alzheimer's disease affects persons with the disease along with their families, caregivers, and communities. Without an effective way to treat or prevent Alzheimer's disease it is estimated that, by the middle of this century, the number of people in the United States affected by the disease will reach or exceed 14 million.

Alzheimer's disease is a progressive, deteriorating, neurological disease. The criteria for diagnosis of the disorder include the presence of a dementia syndrome, an insidious onset with a progressive deteriorating course, and exclusion of all other causes of dementia by history, physical examination, and laboratory tests.

The National Institute of Neurological and Communicative Disorders and Stroke and the Alzheimer's Disease and Related Disorders Association recommend the following criteria in the diagnosis of AD:

❖ The dementia syndrome as established by clinical examination and confirmed by neurological tests.
❖ Deficits in two or more areas of cognition.
❖ Progressive worsening of memory and other cognitive functions.
❖ No disturbance of consciousness.
❖ Onset between the ages of 40 and 90 and most often after age 65.
❖ Absence of systemic disorders or other brain diseases that could account for the progressive deficits in memory or cognition.
  (Raskind and Peskind 1992, 479)

The course of AD can range from three to more than twenty years from the onset of early signs and symptoms. Early signs may be subtle difficulties in memory. Memory loss tends to be more marked for recent events. The person may become disoriented in unfamiliar surroundings and may fail to remember appointments and obligations. As the disease continues to progress, more memory traces become lost or irretrievable and the person may be unable to recognize family members. Personality changes are possible. A common personality change is apathy. Other problems may be anxiety, excessive dependency, the occurrence of angry outbursts, and sleep disorders. In the advanced stages of the disease, a person frequently loses the ability for self-care and personal hygiene. Tremors, seizures, and motor deficits may occur in the late stages of the disease. The later stages may manifest mutism, inability to walk, and loss of bowel and bladder control. Death is usually from pneumonia.

The prevalence of AD is estimated at 10% for persons older than 65 years and 47% for persons older than 85 years (National Institute on Aging and National Institutes of Health 1996). The search for the causes of AD is currently in three areas: genetics, the beta-amyloid protein, and environmental toxins. Research is worldwide. The genetics studies indicate that there is evidence that AD may be caused by extra copies of genes on chromosome 21. Researchers are working with families who exhibit clear indications of inheritance of a form of AD, identified by genetic mutations on chromosome 14 and 21, called familial Alzheimer's disease (FAD). A gene on chromosome 19 appears to be associated with late-onset forms of AD. This gene is responsible for the production of a cholesterol-transporting protein called apolipoprotein E (ApoE). It has been found that inheriting certain forms of ApoE or ApoE4 may increase a person's risk for Alzheimer's disease. Those persons who carry two copies of ApoE4 are more likely to get AD than those persons with one copy of ApoE4 (National Institute on Aging and National Institutes of Health 1996).

The plaques in the brains of people with AD are composed of beta-amyloid protein. It is not clear whether the deposits of beta-amyloid protein are the cause or the result of AD. Researchers are exploring the way beta-amyloid protein originates from the amyloid precursor protein (APP) and is processed or deposited. While amyloid is a primary component of plaques, other proteins also are deposited in the brains of people with AD. In other dementing diseases, such as Creutzfeldt-Jakob disease, a protein known as prion protein is deposited into plaques in the brain. Like beta-amyloid, this prion protein is toxic to brain cells. Researchers are also studying the role of tau, a normal brain protein that is the major component of the neurofibrillary tangles found in AD. Tau processing may serve as a target for the development of new therapies to treat the disease.

Environmental toxins are also a source of inquiry for the causes of AD. Under study as a potential risk factor for AD is history of head trauma. However, history of head trauma was found in fewer than 25% of AD patients. Other environmental toxins under study include water pollution and diet.

The National Advisory Panel on Alzheimer's Disease publishes an annual report on Alzheimer's disease research and recommendations for further study. The following recommendations were presented in 1996:

❖ Specific research should be directed toward exploring a wider variety of living situations for people with Alzheimer's disease and related disorders and the effects on function and quality of life associated with these varied situations.

❖ Research on support services for people with Alzheimer's disease and related disorders and their families (e.g., respite care) needs to address the issue of "dose-response," including better quantification of both elements, the services provided, and the effects achieved.

❖ State and federal governments should adopt uniform language to clearly describe for the public residential-care levels of long-term care services and definitions of residential care based on the type of long-term care services provided.

❖ Appropriate assessment of the individual resident's needs (which does not place an unreasonable burden on staff and facilities) should be required before entry into all levels of care in the long-term care system, whether publicly or privately financed.

❖ There should be created a centralized national database on home- and community-based care capable of generating information to compare quality and cost effectiveness across all types of long-term care.

❖ More work is needed to establish actuarially sound reimbursement rates based on the real financial risks presented by clients with dementia.

❖ Work is needed to assess the relative effectiveness of alternative approaches to long-term care (e.g., assisted living) for clients with Alzheimer's disease and related disorders (ADRD).

To improve rural care, the following recommendations should be considered:

❖ Provide more training grants to increase the knowledge base and supply of rural practitioners working with people with ADRD and their caregivers.

❖ Provide more demonstration services grants with rigorous evaluation components to community mental health centers, community health centers, and county aging services reaching rural areas to develop, implement, and evaluate multidisciplinary outreach programs for people with dementia and their caregivers.

❖ Establish and evaluate mobile diagnostic and follow-up services coordinated by local health-care providers, with referral to "experts" in remote academic medical centers using innovative technology such as fiber-optic networks.

❖ Research on dementia care should address ways that value differences based on ethnicity, immigration status, race, and religion influence caregivers. Do these factors operate differently in rural settings compared to urban areas? Do these values change over the course of the illness, and are they different among caregivers in various geographic regions? What outcomes are desired by family caregivers in rural settings? What interventions enhance or maintain positive caregiving experiences for rural caregivers? Are they different than for their urban counterparts?

❖ More research is needed on special care units with regard to staff and administrative issues.

❖ Determine which individual elements in programs of caring for people with dementia are most beneficial and cost effective.

❖ More study is needed on separating patients with dementia versus integrated care along the continuum of care settings.

❖ Controlled trials of specialized care are needed.

❖ Innovative use of technology for care and training is needed.

❖ Abuse/exploitation and poor care of residents with dementia in special care units versus traditional nursing homes must be studied.

❖ Focus treatment/residential standards differentially on caregiver groups.

❖ Detect and ameliorate depression, pain, anxiety, etc.

❖ Correspond appropriate levels of care with stage of disease.

❖ More research is needed on dementia care in adult day-care centers with regard to cost effectiveness of adult services, including quality of life for both caregiver/family and client/participant.

❖ More research is needed on dementia care in assisted living with regard to outcomes of assisted living compared to nursing-home care; outcomes of costs of aging in place in assisted living (with additional services provided as needed) compared to transfer to nursing homes; for which residents with dementia is assisted living more appropriate than nursing homes; cost effectiveness of small facilities versus larger ones; effect of regulation on assisted living. (Advisory Panel on Alzheimer's Disease 1996)

Dementia in Parkinson's Disease

A high prevalence of dementia is found in persons with Parkinson's disease. The disease presents, clinically, as memory impairment and slowness in thinking. Estimates of the prevalence of dementia in Parkinson's disease range from 14% to 40% (Raskind and Peskind 1992).

Depression is a common, complicating syndrome in Parkinson's disease. Some studies found as many as 46% of Parkinson's patients had depressive symptoms. Several studies demonstrated that in the central nervous system (CNS) serotonergic systems are involved in both depression and dementia, which complicates Parkinson's disease.

Lewy Body Disease

Dementia with Lewy bodies is a broad, generic term that includes the diseases involving cognitive impairment such as diffuse Lewy body disease, Lewy body dementia, and senile dementia of the Lewy body type. Lewy bodies are abnormal globe-shaped structures or lesions within nerve cells in the brainstem, subcortical nuclei, limbic cortex, and neocortex of some older people with dementia. Lewy bodies are found in cases of persons with dementia exhibiting signs of memory impairment, confusional states, paranoid delusions, and visual and auditory hallucinations. Rigidity is common while tremor is less common. Duration of illness ranges from one year to twenty years with progression to severe dementia, rigidity, mutism, quadriparesis, emaciation, and pneumonia, which is most frequently the cause of death. Neuropathological examination reveals widespread Lewy body degeneration throughout the neocortex, limbic structures, and subcortical nuclei.

Lewy body patients do not meet the criteria for the diagnosis of AD because, when compared to AD patients, they are more cognitively intact at time of referral and they have a shorter history and a shorter survival time. Lewy body patients present clinically with visual hallucinations and other behavioral disturbances. Neuropathological examinations reveal numerous senile plaques present, but the neurofibrillary tangles are minimal for the Lewy body type. Dr. Kenji Kosaka described Dementia of the Lewy Body type in 1978, and currently it is reported to be the second most common form of dementia next to AD (National Institute on Aging and National Institutes of Health 1998).

Dementia-Related Disorders

A diagnosis of Multi-Infarct Dementia requires evidence of at least two independent cerebrovascular accidents as determined by both neurological examination and brain imaging. Dementia resulting from cerebrovascular accidents differs from Alzheimer's disease in that AD presents a progressive deterioration.

Vitamin B_{12} deficiency can cause dementia. A study of predominately African American subjects conducted by Lindenbaum et al. in

1988 found that neuropsychiatric problems secondary to vitamin B_{12} deficiency in the absence of mycrocytic anemia may be common and reversible. The study found frequent improvement in cognitive impairment and other behavioral problems following administration of vitamin B_{12} (Raskind and Peskind 1992).

Hypothyroidism can also cause dementia accompanied by irritability, paranoid ideation, and depression. There is evidence that dementia due to hypothyroidism is reversible (Raskind and Peskind 1992).

Dementia and AIDS

HIV-infected patients do not always have dementia clinically. However, about two-thirds of all AIDS patients develop clinical evidence of a neurodegenerative disorder termed "AIDS dementia complex." Elderly persons with HIV infection usually have a history of male homosexual activity or were infected with contaminated blood products. Intravenous drug use is rare among the older population (Raskind and Peskind 1992).

Depression

Depression in patients with dementia is difficult to diagnosis but it has received more attention. A careful history and clinical examination can accurately diagnose depression. Depressive signs and symptoms are common in persons with Alzheimer's disease with a 23% prevalence of depression in AD patients (Raskind and Peskind 1992). Depression in AD patients can affect functional impairment. If treatment improves, functioning and mood behavioral problems lessen.

A depressive disorder can complicate the Alzheimer's disorder. In one study, depressed elderly persons reported memory problems more often than did non-depressed elderly persons, and depressed elderly persons reported indecisiveness, impaired concentration, and mental slowing more frequently than did demented persons (Raskind and Peskind 1992).

Depression in older adults is estimated to affect more than 5% of adults ages 65 and older, but epidemiological evidence has challenged the once-prevailing view that depressive illnesses are more common in those older than 65 years (Raskind and Peskind 1992).

There is greater risk of developing depression for women than for men. Among men, the estimates range from 0.5% to 1.5% for ages 18 to 90 years. Women are 1.5 times more likely to develop major depressive disorders. There is some evidence that, after the seventh decade of life, there is a reversal in the male and female ratio. There is evidence that risk for women declines after age 69. Swedish data indicate that women born after World War II have an increased risk of depressive illness (Anthony and Aboraya 1992).

There is evidence that age-related physical diseases cause depression. Included are cardiovascular diseases, metabolic disorders, and degenerative diseases. Depression symptoms may develop as part of the disease process, but there is also evidence that severe illness may cause depressive symptoms. Family history is associated with the occurrence of depressive disorders in adulthood. Social losses are associated with depression—specifically being separated or divorced, being unemployed, or failing to complete twelve years of schooling (Anthony and Aboraya 1992).

Alcohol and Drug Abuse

Alcohol and drug abuse involve the use of alcohol, barbiturates, tranquilizers, marijuana, cocaine, and other regulated substances. The literature offers little information on late-life drug abuse or dependence. Abuse of prescription medications rather than abuse of illegal drugs is more common in older adults. Late-life substance abuse has been attributed to social losses and stress. Alcohol abuse in older adults is described as being either early onset, intermittent, or reactive alcohol abuse.

Early onset refers to older persons who begin abusing alcohol late in life. Intermittent abusers are occasional abusers, and reactive abusers are those persons who began the use of alcohol following a life crisis such as the death of a spouse. Pain, insomnia, anxiety, and depression may increase the use of substances in an effort to self-medicate. Other risk factors include social isolation and family collusion. Family members may encourage the use of drugs in an effort to help ease pain or discomfort.

Drug and alcohol abuse is under-identified, under-reported, and under-treated in older persons. Frequently, older persons are not working or driving and alcohol abuse is undetected. Family members may regard the use of alcohol as being embarrassing or as one of the few enjoyments left to the older person. Physicians may misdiagnose the

Table 7.2 Prevalence and Ages of Women and Men Who Abuse Alcohol

Ages	% of Women	% of Men
Total	2.3	6.0
30–44	1.1	6.2
45–64	0.3	4.0
65 and Older	0.3	1.8

Source: Anthony and Aboraya, 1992

signs of abuse as symptoms of failing physical or mental health. It is estimated that about 2.8% of adults can be described as currently active alcohol abusers. The prevalence and ages of men and women who abuse alcohol are described in table 7.2.

In Canada, about 11% of adults older than age 60 have drinking problems. In contrast, in China 3.2% abuse alcohol. About 20% of Canadian men ages 65 and older have a history of current or past abuse, while in Taiwan 6% of men have a history of abuse. Risk factors for alcohol abuse in later life include a family history of alcoholism, marital crisis, loose or weakening social ties, and socially disintegrated environments such as poverty or hostility.

In the last decade, moderate use of alcohol (up to two drinks a day) has been suggested to lower the risk of coronary heart disease in men. Studies of reactive drinking in response to stress and as a coping mechanism offer mixed scientific results. Retirement seems to have little impact on alcohol consumption (Borgatta, Montgomery, and Borgatta 1982). Coping studies show mixed results. Some studies find that alcohol is not used as a coping mechanism for life stresses; others find that problem drinkers were more likely to have negative life experiences such as poverty, poor health, and social isolation. Atkinson, Ganzini, and Bernstein (1992) predict a threefold to fourfold increase in alcohol abuse in the United States in the next forty years.

Anxiety Disorders

The 1980s are described as the decade of anxiety (Sheikh 1992). Studies of anxiety received a great deal of attention in the past decade. Between 10% and 20% of older adults experience clinically significant symptoms of anxiety. Sheikh defines anxiety as "a normal human emotion associated with a subjective sense of apprehension or nervousness about some future event" (1992, 410). When this emotion becomes excessive it is considered morbid. Anxiety disorder refers to a constellation of symptoms. Anxiety disorders include phobias, social phobias, agoraphobia, panic disorder, obsessive-compulsive disorder, and generalized anxiety disorder. Panic disorders manifest themselves by somatic and cognitive symptoms such as palpitations, shortness of breath, chest pain, sweating, hot and cold flashes, fear of dying, fear of losing control, and fear of going insane. Panic attacks can occur unexpectedly or in certain situations. Panic disorder is chronic, with frequent recurrences and remissions.

Social phobia is characterized by persistent fear of one or more social situations such as public speaking, inability to eat in the presence of others, and being unable to urinate in a public lavatory. Evidence suggests that the disorder is chronic and persists in old age.

Simple phobia is a persistent fear of a stimulus (object or situation). Examples of simple phobias include fear of dogs, snakes, insects, closed spaces, flying, heights, or fear of victimization of crime.

Obsessive-Compulsive Disorder

Sheikh states "obsessive-compulsive disorder is characterized by recurrent obsessions or compulsions sufficiently severe to cause marked distress or dysfunction in occupational or personal matters. Obsessions are ideas, thoughts, impulses, or images that are experienced as senseless or intrusive and persist despite attempts to suppress them" (1992, 415).

Common obsessions are repetitive thoughts such as fear of contamination by germs or concerns about offending someone. Compulsions are repetitive behaviors performed in response to an obsession. The compulsive behavior is designed to avert anxiety and reduce tension. Examples of compulsive behaviors include hand washing, counting, checking, and touching.

Generalized Anxiety Disorder

Generalized anxiety disorder can be diagnosed when there are symptoms of excessive or unrealistic anxiety on most days, for six months or more. A diagnosis of anxiety by clinical assessment should include a physical examination and a detailed mental status examination. Anxiety scales are useful in diagnosing anxiety disorder, and the most popular is the Hamilton Anxiety Rating Scale (HARS), which measures the severity of anxiety in patients diagnosed with anxiety disorder. The occurrence of depression and anxiety is common in older adults. As many as 80% of depressed patients manifest symptoms of anxiety and 35% of anxious persons experience depression. This mixed-symptom situation is found quite frequently in the elderly.

The effect of anxiety on physical health is not known. Evidence exists that high anxiety predisposes occurrence of myocardial infarction in older men (Sheikh 1992). Anxiety is associated with high blood pressure, kidney or bladder disease, heart trouble, stomach ulcers, hardening of the arteries, stroke, asthma, and diabetes. Cause and effect require further studies.

Dietary causes of anxiety are linked to caffeine consumption. Drug-related causes of anxiety are a common side effect of neuroleptics or over-the-counter drugs such as pseudoephedrine, which is common in cold medicines. Alcohol withdrawal is a cause of anxiety, and sedative withdrawal is underestimated as a cause of anxiety. Drugs that cause anxiety symptoms are amphetamines, bronchodilators, and calcium blockers such as verapamil.

Anxiety disorders are treated with psychological and/or pharmacological interventions. Psychological treatments include relaxation training and cognitive restructuring. Cognitive behavior therapy is effective

Table 7.3 Symptoms of Generalized Anxiety Disorder

Motor tension	Trembling, muscle tension, restlessness
Vigilance and scanning	Feeling on edge, exaggerated startle response, difficulty concentrating, insomnia, irritability
Hyperactivity	Shortness of breath, rapid heart rate, sweating or cold clammy hands, dry mouth, dizziness, digestive disturbances, hot flashes or chills, frequent urination, trouble swallowing

Source: Sheikh, 1992

in panic disorder. Pharmacological treatments include the use of benzodiazepines like diazepam or chlordiazepoxide. Buspirone is an anxiolytic with partial serontonin-agonist properties that are reported to be tolerated well by geriatric patients and effective for relief of anxiety symptoms. Antidepressants are the treatment of choice for the mixed anxiety-depression syndromes. Imipramine has been shown to be effective (Salzman and Nevis-Olesen 1992). There is a need for research on causes and treatments of anxiety disorders and the aged. It is essential for professionals to recognize symptoms of anxiety and to provide interventions. See Appendix A for a Generalized Anxiety Disorder Self-Test.

Summary

Scientists worldwide study the epidemiology (incidence and prevalence) of mental and physical disease common to older persons. Research is being conducted for causes and therapeutic interventions in Alzheimer's disease, depression, alcoholism, and anxiety disorders. Older persons are enjoying better health and increased years of life. The leading causes of mortality for older men and older women are diseases of the heart, cancer, and cerebrovascular diseases. Mental health problems of the older population are influenced by social structures such as family, community and institutional care, ethnic and cultural differences, and socioeconomic status. Prevalent mental health problems for older persons are Alzheimer's disease or related dementias, depression, anxiety disorders, drug abuse, and alcoholism. Increased numbers of older persons who have chronic illnesses will be a burden to health-care systems. Research is essential to find interventions for the physical and mental illnesses commonly found in older persons, to control costs, and to improve quality of life in old age.

References

Advisory Panel on Alzheimer's Disease. 1996. *Alzheimer's disease and related dementias: Acute and long term care services.* NIH Pub. No. 96–4136. Washington, D.C.: GPO.

Alzheimer's Association. 2000. Online: http://www.alz.org/hc/overview/stats.htm

Anthony, J. C., and A. Aboraya. 1992. The epidemiology of selected mental disorders in later life. In *Handbook of mental health and aging,* edited by J. E. Birren, R. B. Sloane, and G. D. Cohen. 2nd ed. San Diego, Calif.: Academic Press.

Atkinson, R. M., L. Ganzini, and M. J. Bernstein. 1992. Alcohol. In *Handbook of mental health and aging*, edited by J. E. Birren, R. B. Sloane, and G. D. Cohen. 2nd ed. San Diego, Calif.: Academic Press.

Birren, J. E., R. B. Sloane, and G. D. Cohen, eds. 1992. *Handbook of mental health and aging*. 2nd ed. San Diego, Calif.: Academic Press.

Borgatta, E. F., R. J. V. Montgomery, and M. L. Borgatta. 1982. Alcohol use and abuse, life crisis events, and the elderly. In *Alcoholism and aging: An annotated bibliography and review*, edited by Nancy J. Osgood, Helen E. Wood, and Iris A. Parham. 1995. Westport, Conn.: Greenwood Press.

Choe, Ehn Hyun. 1989. *Population Aging in the Republic of Korea*. UNESCAP Asian Population Studies Series No. 97. In addition, as reported to the World Health Organization.

Hooyman, N., and H. A. Kiyak. 1996. *Social gerontology: A multidisciplinary perspective*. 4th ed. Boston: Allyn and Bacon.

Koster, J., and J. Prather. 1998. *Global aging report: Aging everywhere*. Washington, D.C.: AARP.

National Institute on Aging and National Institutes of Health. 1996. *Progress report on Alzheimer's disease*. NIH Publication No. 96–4137. Washington, D.C.: Department of Health and Human Services, Public Health Service, and National Institutes of Health.

National Institute on Aging and National Institutes of Health. 1998. *Connections: Newsletter published by the Alzheimer's Disease Education and Referral Center* 7 (2) (fall): 1–6.

National Institutes of Health and National Institute on Aging. 1993. *In search of the secrets of aging*. NIH Publication No. 93–2756. Washington, D.C.: Department of Health and Human Services, Public Health Service, and National Institutes of Health.

Raskind, M. A., and E. R. Peskind. 1992. Alzheimer's disease and other dementing disorders. In *Handbook of mental health and aging*, edited by J. E. Birren, R. B. Sloane, and G. D. Cohen. 2nd ed. San Diego, Calif.: Academic Press.

Salzman, C., and J. Nevis-Olesen. 1992. Psychopharmacologic treatment. In *Handbook of mental health and aging*, edited by J. E. Birren, R. B. Sloane, and G. D. Cohen. 2nd ed. San Diego, Calif.: Academic Press.

Sheikh, J. I. 1992. Anxiety and its disorders in old age. In *Handbook of mental health and aging*, edited by J. E. Birren, R. B. Sloane, and G. D. Cohen. 2nd ed. San Diego, Calif.: Academic Press.

U.S. Bureau of the Census, International Population Reports. 1992. *An aging world II.* P25, 92–3. Washington, D.C.: GPO.

CHAPTER EIGHT

Attitudes about Aging

Attitudes about aging and the aged influence program development, policy issues, and service delivery. Globally there are cultural differences in attitudes toward the aged. Negative attitudes toward old men and old women are more common in Western cultures. Respect and admiration for older persons are traditional in Eastern cultures. The concept of *Xaio,* or filial piety, is an Eastern concept and it refers to respect and responsibility for elders. Negative and positive attitudes toward old age are found in literature, art, history, and religion. In this book, the following definitions are used:

- ❖ *Attitude* is defined as a manner of thinking, acting, or feeling that shows one's disposition or opinion (Geralnik 1974).
- ❖ *Stereotype* is defined as a fixed or conventional notion or conception of a person, group, or idea held by a number of people and allowing for no individuality or critical judgment (Geralnik 1974).
- ❖ *Ageism* is defined as a negative attitude toward older persons.
- ❖ *Gerontophobia* is defined as fear of aging.

Historically, literature and art of ageism portray gerontophobia. Thomas Cole's (1842) series of paintings, *The Voyage of Life,* depicts human lifetime as a journey down a river. Childhood and youth are painted as voyages of beauty while adulthood and old age is painted as a voyage of darkness. Childhood and youth are colorful and bright, suggesting beauty and hope. Manhood, or middle age, is depicted by storms and turbulence while old age is depicted by night, darkness, and gloom. There are other suggestions of ageism in literature. The character of Scrooge in Dickens's 1843 classic, *A Christmas Carol,* is a miserly, old man.

The increase of the older population is considered a social problem. If aging is a state of dependency, then an increasing number of dependent older adults suggests intergenerational conflict. Ageist ideology represents aging as a time of dependency and disengagement, a withdrawal from life.

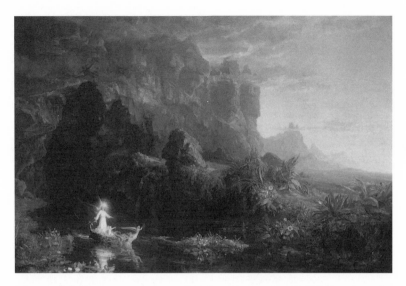

Thomas Cole (American, 1801–1848), The Voyage of Life: Childhood, *1842, oil on canvas, 52 7/8 x 77 7/8 in.* Ailsa Mellon Bruce Fund. Photograph © Board of Trustees, National Gallery of Art, Washington, D.C.

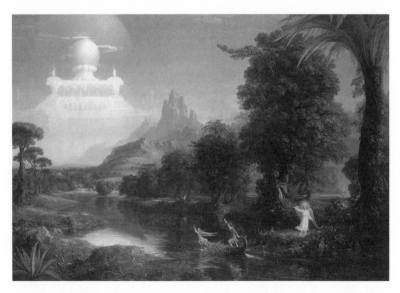

Thomas Cole (American, 1801–1848), The Voyage of Life: Youth, *1842, oil on canvas, 52 7/8 x 76 3/4 in.* Ailsa Mellon Bruce Fund. Photograph © Board of Trustees, National Gallery of Art, Washington, D.C.

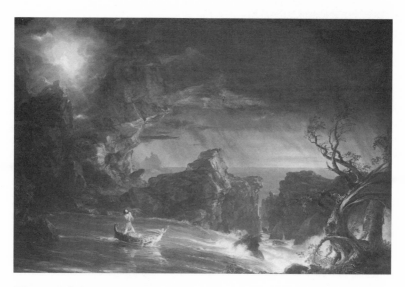

Thomas Cole (American, 1801–1848), The Voyage of Life: Manhood, *1842, oil on canvas, 52 7/8 x 79 3/4 in.* Ailsa Mellon Bruce Fund. Photograph © Board of Trustees, National Gallery of Art, Washington, D.C.

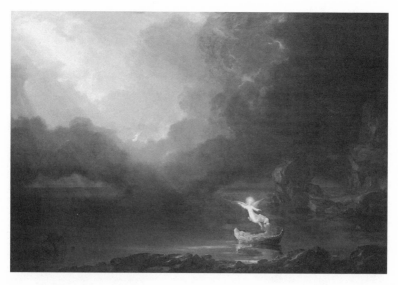

Thomas Cole (American, 1801–1848), The Voyage of Life: Old Age, *1842, oil on canvas, 52 1/2 x 77 1/4 in.* Ailsa Mellon Bruce Fund. Photograph © Board of Trustees, National Gallery of Art, Washington, D.C.

Another perspective by Calasanti (1999) uses the term "age blindness." She argues that age blindness reinforces systems of oppression and that, with this blindness, we adopt a mid-life perspective in a way that argues that old people are acceptable only if they are like young people. She argues that this idea is similar to stating that women who behave like men are okay and black people are acceptable if they are like white people. She proposes that there is a double standard of aging in which women are considered old sooner than men.

Myths and Stereotypes about Aging

Myths and stereotypes about aging influence policy and social planning for older adults. Sociological theories of disengagement and activity strongly influenced the development of senior centers, the boom in construction of nursing homes, and the passage of the Older Americans Act. Social policies supporting nursing-home construction were based on a disengagement perspective, while the activity theory supported construction of senior centers, congregate meal programs, and the employment programs of the Older Americans Act.

Ageism is obvious in the use of the terms *productive aging* or *successful aging*. Working and active older persons are described as successful agers. Palmore's study (1993) found negative stereotypes associated with aging including illness, impotency, ugliness, mental decline, mental illness, uselessness, isolation, poverty, and depression. Since 1950 attitudes have changed and are becoming more positive (Barrow 1996) but remain predominately negative.

Stereotyping in recent years was derived from *biomedicalization*— which focuses on the less healthy, the frail, and the problems of aging persons—and what Binstock refers to as *compassionate stereotyping* (Barrow 1996). This kind of negativism describes older persons as being disadvantaged—either socially, psychologically, or economically. Myths about old people and old age are common but ten popular myths were selected.

- ❖ Myth #1   Older persons are greedy geezers.
- ❖ Myth #2   Older persons are poor.
- ❖ Myth #3   Older persons are lonely and sad.
- ❖ Myth #4   Older persons are not sexual.
- ❖ Myth #5   Older persons are unattractive.

❖ Myth #6   Older persons want to be only with older persons.
❖ Myth #7   Older persons do not keep up with new ideas.
❖ Myth #8   Older persons are not involved in communities.
❖ Myth #9   Older persons are abandoned by their families.
❖ Myth #10   Older persons are sick and depressed.

Myth #1   Older persons are greedy geezers.

Older adults want more benefits but do not want to support young people. This myth contributes to the belief that older persons are greedy. Older adults contributed to the social and economic well-being of the society in which they have lived, worked, and raised families. At a time when retirement income is fixed and costs continue to rise, the older person is at risk of economic disadvantage. Particular concerns are the high costs of health-care coverage and medication costs. In the United States, there has been strong resistance to providing federal or state financial assistance for the cost of medications. It is possible that this resistance can be attributed to the "greedy geezer" belief.

Myth #2   Older persons are poor.

While some older persons are poor, the majority are financially better off than at any other time in history. In 1992, 12.9% of persons older than age 65 were living with incomes below the poverty threshold. In the past fifty years, the economic situation of older persons improved (Kart 1997). Substantial increases in Social Security benefits, the growth of private pension plans, improvements of health-insurance programs, widespread property tax relief, and more local programs for older persons have contributed to the improvement in the economic well-being of older persons.

The economic situation of older persons has improved considerably. About three of four older persons own their own homes in the United States, while in Australia more than 75% of older persons own their own homes. In underdeveloped countries, poverty of older persons is still a problem and homelessness of older adults is a serious issue. Older women have the highest rates of poverty.

Myth #3   Older persons are lonely and sad.

The myth that older people are lonely and sad is compassionate stereotyping. This belief adds to the fears of aging. Most older people are not lonely and sad. Older persons are involved with community organizations, families, and a variety of activities from sports to volunteerism. Americans see leisure time as the best aspect of growing old (AARP 1995). Americans reported they enjoy the freedom and independence of the later years, but most Americans have misconceptions that older people are poor, lonely, bored, and often angry. The AARP study found a relationship between those who had a low level of knowledge about aging and very negative stereotypes of aging and the elderly.

Myth #4   Older persons are not sexual.

Older persons describe themselves as no longer sexual and believe that sex is not for the old. This myth is self-fulfilling. Expressions of sexuality by older persons may be embarrassing for adult children and health professionals. Studies indicate that older men and women who are in reasonably good health have no age-related decline in sexual interest (Kart 1997). If they were sexually active in earlier years, they will remain sexually active in later years. Some decline is attributed to older people's acceptance of society's attitudes that the aging years are sexless years. Some older persons are embarrassed about having sexual interests. Older people who cannot maintain the sexual experiences of youth

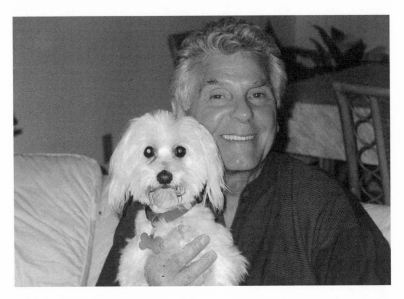

Pets can bring comfort and joy.

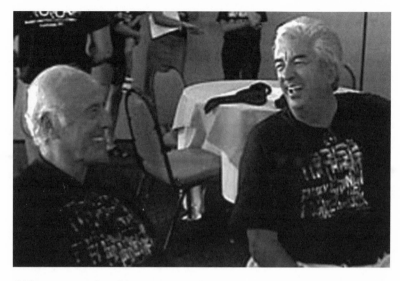

Older men enjoy friendships.

attribute these changes to impotence (Kart 1997). Kart (1997) proposes that some of the blame for the lack of sexual functioning and sexual interest in later years should be attributed to health professionals who are not helping older people to appreciate the importance of sexuality in the later years.

Myth #5   Older persons are unattractive.

Greeting cards depict societal negative attitudes about aging with cards that describe those who are having 40- or 50-year birthdays as being "over the hill." Black decorations for parties for those who reach 50 years of age and jokes about physical and sexual decline are common. The media, the movies, and the fashion industry can take responsibility for perpetuating the magic of youth as beautiful. Older women are portrayed as ugly, asexual, wrinkled, etc. Women traditionally value themselves as beautiful according to their attractiveness to men. Some women torture and change their bodies in the name of beauty. When they age and are no longer attractive to men, the prospect of growing old can be frightening.

Women are trained to be ageist. Women have learned not to value themselves if they are not valued by men. The common story of the older husband who leaves his wife for a younger woman perpetuates the fear of aging for women. The cosmetic industry, in helping women to avoid aging, is said to be one of the fastest-growing industries in America. Men also are seen as not attractive as they age. Baldness and loss of physical strength are of serious concern. Older adults maintain their beauty and vigor well into old age as is evident in movie stars who are considered attractive such as Omar Sharif and Sophia Loren.

Myth #6   Older persons want to be only with other older persons.

The belief that older persons do not want to be with young people is a common misconception. Are we an age-segregated society in which older persons live in age-segregated communities with golf courses, tennis courts, and a variety of leisure activities? No; rather, most older adults *age in place* and remain in the communities where they have been most of their lives. Only 3% to 5% of older persons move to retirement communities (Hooyman and Kiyak 1996). However, lack of services and assistance in some communities often forces older persons to move into communities in which assistance is available for them. The lower cost of living in some states also attracts older people to certain regions.

Myth #7   Older persons do not keep up with new ideas.

Our society values people who work and are productive. New technology tends to make skills and knowledge obsolete. Most people of all ages are struggling to keep up to date with the changes in communication technology. Older adults are described as "out of it," not knowledgeable in the use of new technology, and resistant to learning the use of new equipment. Employers seek younger persons in the work force while older persons are devalued, discounted, and often encouraged to retire. Contrary to this myth, 50% of buyers of personal computers are older than 50 years. With training, older people can keep pace on the "information highway" (Barrow 1996).

Studies of older persons indicate that mental abilities do not decline and, in fact, there is little decline in intelligence scores over the years. Older people are as capable as younger people of learning new tasks. Older persons have created masterpieces in art and music in their later years. Verdi composed his opera *Falstaff* when he was age 80 years, and

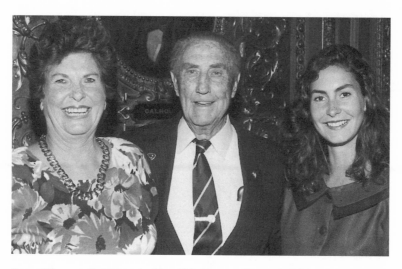

Strom Thurmond, 100 years old, a U.S. Senator for nearly fifty years, supported Fulbright scholars.

Georgia O'Keeffe remained a world-renowned painter in her eighties. Senator Strom Thurmond, the U.S. Senator from South Carolina, remained an active member of Congress till his hundreth birthday.

Myth #8   Older persons are not involved in communities.

The myth that most older persons are not interested in their communities and do not support programs for the young creates conflict between generations. Older adults are a major force in volunteerism in America, Australia, and most developed countries. In underdeveloped countries, older adults provide childcare and support for their working adult children. In Nigeria, older women are childbirth attendants, and in China older women manage the household, allowing younger women to participate in the workforce (Sadik 1996). Older adults are quite involved in volunteerism, and from 40% to 50% of older persons are active members of religious organizations (Koenig 1997).

Myth #9   Older persons are abandoned by their families.

The Walton family is an idealized American family myth. The extended family living together in the "good old days" is a myth. Those families rarely existed because life expectancy in the early 1900s was in the fifties. In the 1800s, the median age was 18 years of age. There is a myth that the American nuclear family is isolated from its older family members. However, the major responsibility for aged relatives still remains with American families. The change in the family is that families are no longer the only means of support for older persons. Shanas (1980) found that more than 50% of people older than 65 are members of four-generation families. Most older people live near but not with their children. Most older people prefer not to live with their children. In the National Survey of Families and Households (1994), only 7% of Americans ages 55 and older with a surviving parent reported that the parent was living with them. Hispanic and Asian widows are more likely to be living with family members than white and African American widows. Most older people do not end their lives in nursing homes. Only 5% of older Americans reside in institutions, which means that 95% live at home (Kart 1997).

Myth #10   Older persons are sick and depressed.
While many older adults have chronic health conditions that require treatment, more and more older people are healthy and active. Senior Olympics and senior involvement in all sports have largely dispelled this myth. Certainly John Glenn's trip at age 77 aboard the space shuttle in 1999 was an indicator of the abilities of a fit older person. More and more older people are involved in tennis, jogging, aerobics, walking, and bicycling as well as other sports. In addition, physical exercise has been shown to improve well-being even when started as late in life as the eighties (Schulz-Aellen 1997).

Depression is a common mental health problem among older persons, but research evidence suggests that depression is a lifelong condition. Older persons who suffer from depression have most likely suffered from depression in other periods of their lives. Additionally, treatment for depression in older adults has high success rates. Psychopharmacology and psychological treatment are effective treatments. Unfortunately, however, many cases of depression are undiagnosed due to stereotypical attitudes that being old and being depressed are synonymous. Physicians may attribute symptoms of depression to aging changes. New evidence indicates that some physical illnesses are causal for depression (Anthony and Aboraya 1992).

Attitudes of the Young about the Old and Aging

What are the attitudes of young people toward the old and toward aging? What do adolescents think about aging? What are some of the factors that influence negative or positive attitudes?

Respect for the old in American society is not common. Fear of aging and its financial and social burdens permeates American attitudes. Gerontologist Ken Dychtwald argues that more young people believe in UFOs (Unidentified Flying Objects) than in Social Security (Dychtwald 1998).

Children's attitudes about aging and older adults were investigated using an instrument called Children's Views on Aging, which was designed to assess school-age children's attitudes toward older adults and aging (Newman, Faux, and Larimer 1997). The study reports that children's perceptions about aging and older adults are not as negative as adults believe. They state that children are positively affected by interactions with older adults, describe physical signs of aging without judgment, but respond negatively to some of the unpleasant conditions associated with aging.

Other studies report that children's attitudes today are more positive than they were twenty or thirty years ago and that ageist attitudes are taught early, even in fairy tales in which witches are old, ugly, and frightening. More recently, children's books emphasize relationships between grandparents and grandchildren. School-age children were found to have positive attitudes toward older persons when asked to choose descriptive adjectives to apply to them, such as an older person is mean or gentle, good or bad, and weak or strong. They found that the children described the personality traits of the older person more positively but the physical traits more negatively. Another study of five-year-old children who visited nursing-home patients had more negative attitudes toward older persons. Researchers urged that those contacts should be balanced with contact with healthy and active older persons (Barrow 1996).

An educational intervention was used to assess the attitudes and knowledge of students ages 17 and 18 in Australia, using Palmore's Facts on Aging Quiz. The results revealed that students had low knowledge of older people and held negative attitudes about aging (pre-intervention scores). Post-intervention, students still held negative attitudes toward older people and there was little change in their attitudes following the intervention program (Scott, Minichiello, and Browning 1998).

Barrow (1996) studied the attitudes of college students by using a word association test. The analysis of the study was grouped into three categories: social, psychological, and physical. A significant finding of the study was that college students were most concerned with the change in physical appearance and capabilities of older persons. Many responded with words that described physical decline.

In the study, the most frequent physical word responses to the word "aged" were: wrinkled, gray hair, slow, less energy, helpless, weak, deterioration, body broken down, over the hill, washed up, death, dying, walkers, canes, handicapped, arthritis, bad back, hospitals, sick, fragile, stooped, ugly, and no teeth.

The most frequent social responses to the word "aged" were: bad drivers, poor, interesting life stories, family, grandchildren, bingo, rich, overworked, retirement, and caretakers.

Psychological responses were: wise, lonely, experienced, shrieking, fear of death, racist, inner conflicts, no spirit, enraged, smart, Alzheimer's, set in ways, closed-minded, opinionated, and giving.

Young people describe older people as being depressed, sick, and unhappy. Older people see themselves as having fewer problems than younger people. Another study explored the attitudes of college students who were studying business, psychology, nursing, and occupational therapy to determine if there were differences among them. Few differences were found across majors (Mosher-Ashley and Ball 1999).

Attitudes of Professionals about the Old and Aging

Health-care professionals are reported to have negative attitudes about older persons. Clinical psychologists considered older depressed clients less ideal than younger clients with the same symptoms, and medical students were reluctant to work with older patients (Barrow 1996). Gatz and Pearson (1988) found that prevalent negative attitudes exist in the health-care field. Educational institutions may be responsible for negative attitudes toward older persons. Santos and VandenBos (1982) found that few graduate programs in the social sciences offer training in gerontology. Whitbourne and Hulicka (1990) analyzed 139 psychology textbooks for evidence of ageism. Written over the course of forty years, the texts fail to mention differences in normal aging and pathological aging, focus on the problems of aging, and describe older adults from a deficit perspective.

Professional groups such as the Association for Gerontology Education in Social Work (AGE-SW) are concerned about the shortage of social workers in the field of aging. New projects by the Council on Social Work Education and the Hartford Foundation Geriatric Faculty Scholars Initiative are underway to foster education in geriatric social work.

The media is negative in its portrayal of older persons. Older persons in television programs are often portrayed as being bent, gray-haired, frail, and forgetful. Older women behave foolishly, dress inappropriately, or wear outdated clothes. Stereotypic images of the elderly in advertising are of frail older persons with physical problems who need diapers, denture powders, medicine, or nutritional supplements.

In an analysis of humorous birthday cards, researchers found that of 496 birthday cards, 39% focused on aging. The cards were coded for negative or positive attitudes about aging. The most frequent themes were appearance, sexuality, concealment of age, and declining abilities. Coders judged more messages as negative than positive (Demos and Jache 1980).

From the political scene, it seems that legislators in state and federal government have either negative attitudes or compassionate (negative) attitudes about the elderly. A study by Lumomudrov found that legislators who were on committees on aging did not express negative stereotypes but held compassionate negative views about elderly constituents (Kart 1997).

Training in gerontology is lacking in most professions. Geriatric training in most medical schools for physicians and psychiatrists remains low (Nathanson and Tirrito 1998). In a study of medical students, a change in attitude was noted after geriatric training. A negative attitude toward the elderly affects treatment and care (Baiyewu et al. 1997). Schools of social work, public health, and other health professions offer aging courses as elective courses rather than as required courses. Schools of business, management, hotel management, politics, engineering, and architecture are ignoring demographics that predict that large numbers of older persons, globally, will need services.

Attitudes of the Old about Being Old and Aging

What do older persons think of themselves? How old is old? What are the fears and concerns of the aged? Gerontologists believe that compassionate stereotyping perpetuates dependency and low self-esteem (Barrow 1996). Self-esteem affects an individual psychologically. Studies of identity find that older people do not see themselves as old. Older persons report being unable to realize their chronological age with comments such as, "I feel as if I am 40 years of age even though I know I am 90 years of age." A Toronto study describes "the ageless self as: it is our bodies getting old, not us. You don't feel any different but other people see you as older" (Barrow 1996).

Negative attitudes of older persons about getting old are detrimental to their well-being and become self-fulfilling prophecies. A study that measured fear of aging and found that older persons who did not fear aging felt good about themselves and their lives while those persons who were fearful of aging did not have a good personal sense of well-being (Barrow 1996). Negative stereotypes about aging contribute to the view that older persons are less valuable members of society.

The self-fulfilling prophecy is evident in a study of older people in Hong Kong. More than 90% perceived themselves as senile, declining in the five senses, weak in strength, and losing interest in sex. More than half of the aged respondents agreed that older people often feel miserable and were not receptive to changes. About one-third agreed that elders are often bored and are easily irritated. Both the aged and the young agreed that the older persons learned more slowly and were isolated and lonely. Chow (1999) concluded that members of the present generation of elders have the impression that they are physically weak, stubborn in character, economically dependent, and socially isolated. Chow proposes that the role and status of elders has changed and that, while filial piety still exists, elders are less valued because they no longer occupy important positions.

Americans perceive health, isolation, and financial problems as aging problems. When asked to respond to a list of thirteen items concerning problems of aging, American responses included not enough money, poor health, and loneliness. Persons with less education and higher anxiety expressed more unfounded negative attitudes about aging.

Americans think of old age as beginning in the early sixties. When asked what age the average man or woman becomes old, the responses were that old age begins for men at 63 years and at 62 years for women. Americans are anxious about aging. About one-half of Americans surveyed had anxiety about health, independence, finances, decision-making, or the future. Americans were confident that they would have friends and an active sex life in old age but worried about physical dependence and cognitive dependence (others making decisions for them). Anxiety was related to past experiences, and disenfranchised groups were found to have higher anxiety levels about aging. Fear of financial dependence on children was related to current experience with problems with money and fear of not being able to afford medical care (AARP 1995).

Attitudes of Baby Boomers about Aging

Dychtwald (1998) proposes that baby boomers will change America's attitudes about aging. Baby boomers will age in unprecedented numbers and will have a powerful influence on social and political forces in

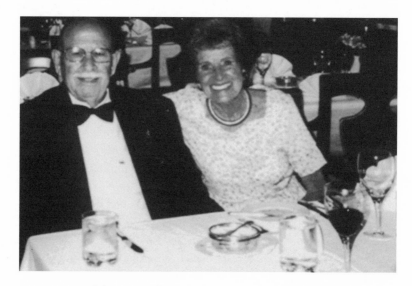

Positive views of the process of aging can improve the outlook for all people as they age.

America. He predicts that markets will change clothing designs, travel accommodations, automobile design, and even investment planning. Aging baby boomers will have resources that were not available to previous cohorts of older persons. Women will have earned incomes independently of their spouses and some baby boomers will not marry. Delayed marriages and high divorce rates of baby boomers have forced some women to manage their lives independently.

Baby boomers will benefit from information and communications technology. They will be computer literate and well-prepared to find information using the Internet. Worldwide, baby boomers are communicating and learning about medicine, health care, and health professionals. Longino (1999) describes self-care via the Internet as a trend that cannot be stopped. Boomers are leading the trends in America and they will insist on quality services in their old age. Old age is changing so that 65 years of age is no longer considered to be old. The baby boomers will change the way Americans and the world perceive aging. The baby boomers changed social patterns in the 1950s, 1970s, and 1990s, and they will challenge aging myths in the next millennium to a more positive image of aging.

Summary

The attitude that the elderly are problem ridden and that increases in the older population is a social problem establishes a negative image of aging and of old people. Negative attitudes perpetuate fear of aging, discrimination, and negative self-images. A change in ageist attitudes is essential for the well-being of all members of society. Ageism perpetuates polarization between the young and the old and intergenerational conflict. Does contemporary society still hold the attitudes reflected in a rhyme from fifteenth- and sixteenth-century German people about the ages of life (Cole 1992)?

> 10 years—a child
> 20 years—a youth
> 30 years—a man
> 40 years—standing still
> 50 years—settled and prosperous
> 60 years—departing

70 years—protect your soul
80 years—the world's fool
90 years—scorn of children
100 years—God have mercy

References

American Association of Retired Persons (AARP). 1995. *Images of aging in America.* Prepared by K. Speas and B. Obenshain. Washington, D.C.: AARP.

Anthony, J. C., and A. Aboraya. 1992. The epidemiology of selected mental disorders in later life. In *Handbook of mental health and aging,* edited by J. E. Birren, R. B. Sloane, and G. D. Cohen. 2nd ed. San Diego, Calif.: Academic Press.

Baiyewu, O., A. F. Bella, J. D. Adeyemi, B. A. Ikuesan, E. A. Bamgboye, and R. O. Jegede. 1997. Attitude to aging among different groups in Nigeria. *International Journal of Aging and Human Development* 44 (4): 283–92.

Barrow, Georgia M. 1996. *Aging, the individual, and society.* 6th ed. Minneapolis/St. Paul, Minn.: West Publishing.

Calasanti, Toni M. 1999. Feminism and gerontology: Not just for women. *Hallym International Journal of Aging* 1 (1): 44–55.

Chow, Nelson. 1999. Diminishing filial piety and the changing role and status of the elders in Hong Kong. *Hallym International Journal of Aging* 1 (1): 67–77.

Cole, Thomas R. 1992. *The journey of life: A cultural history of aging in America.* Cambridge: Cambridge Univ. Press.

Demos, V., and A. Jache. 1980. If you really care: An analysis of attitudes towards aging as expressed in humorous birthday cards. Paper presented at the North Central Sociological Association (NCSA).

Dychtwald, K. 1998. *The middlescence.* Videotape. Emeryville, Calif.: Age Wave.

Gatz, M., and C. G. Pearson. 1988. Ageism revised and the provision of psychological services. *American Psychologist* 43: 184–88.

Geralnik, David, ed. 1974. *Webster's new world dictionary.* 2nd ed. New York: Williams Collins and World Publishing.

Hooyman, N., and H. A. Kiyak. 1996. *Social gerontology: A multidisciplinary perspective.* 4th ed. Boston: Allyn and Bacon.

Kart, Cary S. 1997. *The realities of aging: An introduction to gerontology.* 5th ed. Boston: Allyn and Bacon.

Koenig, H. 1997. *Is religion good for your health? The effects of religion on physical and mental health.* New York: Haworth Press.

Longino, C. F., Jr. 1999. The future population aging in the U.S.A. and Pacific Rim countries: Implications are not always obvious. *Hallym International Journal of Aging* 1 (1): 33–43.

Mosher-Ashley, P. M., and P. Ball. 1999. Attitudes of college students toward elderly persons and their perceptions of themselves at age 75. *Educational Gerontology* (UK) 25 (1): 89–102.

Nathanson, I., and T. Tirrito. 1998. *Gerontological social work: Theory into practice.* New York: Springer Publishing.

Newman, S., R. Faux, and B. Larimer. 1997. Children's views on aging: Their attitudes and values. *Gerontologist* 37: 412–17.

Palmore, E. 1993. United States. *Developments and research on aging: An international handbook.* Westport, Conn.: Greenwood Press.

Sadik, N. 1996. In spite of poverty. The older population builds toward the future. Symposium conducted by the American Association of Retired Persons, the African American Institute, and the UNCHS (habitat), New York.

Santos, John F., and G. R. VandenBos. 1982. *Psychology and the older adult: Challenges for training in the 1980s.* Washington, D.C.: American Psychological Association.

Schulz-Aellen, Marie Francoise. 1997. *Aging and human longevity.* Boston: Birkhauser Boston.

Scott, T., V. Minichiello, and C. Browning. 1998. Secondary school students' knowledge of and attitudes toward older people: Does an education intervention programme make a difference? *Aging and Society* 18: 167–83.

Shanas, E. 1980. Older people and their families: The new pioneers. *Journal of Marriage and Family* 42: 9–14.

Whitbourne, S. K., and I. M. Hulicka. 1990. Ageism in undergraduate psychology texts. *American Psychologist* 45: 1127–36.

CHAPTER NINE

Experiences of Aging for Women, Gay Men and Lesbians, and Ethnic and Minority Older Adults

Women, gay men, lesbians, and ethnic and minority persons deal with aging issues based on their earlier sociocultural experiences. Women, gay men, lesbians, and ethnic and minority older adults are particularly at risk for poverty, poor health, and lack of services and are termed as being in double jeopardy (being a woman and old, being gay and old) or being in triple jeopardy (being a woman, old, and a member of a minority group).

Life expectancy is lower and physical and mental health problems are more prevalent. Sociopsychological issues that affect older women are different from those that affect men. Access to services is an issue for gay men and lesbians and minority groups. Ethnic and minority groups are disenfranchised and discriminated against, and many services are not culturally sensitive or not available for them. Aging is a different experience for ethnic minority groups than for their white counterparts. Gay men and lesbians must adapt to the physical and emotional changes of aging in an environment that is often hostile to them.

Gay Men and Lesbian Older Adults in the United States

Unlike ethnic minorities, women, and racial minorities, gay men and lesbians are not counted in the United States Census. Therefore data on older gay men and lesbian women are sparse. However, Overlooked Opinions, a Chicago polling organization, collects data on gay and lesbian Americans.

In some cities, older gay men and lesbian women will most likely seek services as they age. Concentrations of the lesbian and gay population in the United States are:

1. Manhattan	7. Chicago/Evanston	13. Portland
2. San Francisco	8. Atlanta	14. San Diego
3. Boston/Cambridge	9. Minneapolis	15. Pittsburgh
4. Seattle	10. Marin County, Calif.	
6. Washington, D.C.	12. Santa Monica Bay	

The following demographics describe facts about gay men and lesbians in the United States.

❖ Of all lesbians and gay men, 45.1% and 52.7%, respectively, live in urban areas while 33.1% and 31.7%, respectively, live in the suburbs.

❖ Ten percent of the population of California is lesbian or gay, constituting 12.1% of the lesbian and gay population of the United States. Twenty-seven percent of the population of San Francisco is gay or lesbian.

❖ There are some 9,301 same-sex couples living in New York City, 6,816 in San Francisco, 3,842 in Chicago, and 2,213 in Washington, D.C. (Census officials admit that these figures do not reflect the true number of same-sex couples living together.)

❖ As of 1989, an estimated 15,000 to 20,000 postoperative male-to-female transsexuals were living in the United States.

❖ More than a substantial percentage of lesbians (82%) and gay men (69%) had some college training.

❖ More than 90% of lesbians and 92.9% of gay men were registered to vote in the last presidential election.

❖ Thirty-six percent of lesbian and gay Americans live in households earning $50,000 or more, and 7% live in households earning $100,000 or more.

❖ The average household income for lesbians in the United States is estimated at $45,927, and for gay men it is estimated to be $51,325; the average household income in the United States in 1990 was $36,520.

❖ Between 1988 and 1991, gay men and lesbians bought 5,925,000 home computers.

❖ In 1988, 73% of gay men and lesbians took at least one airline trip while the national average was 17.4%.

❖ More than 50% of lesbians reported being abused by their female partner.

❖ Between 350,000 and 650,000 gay men in the United States are victims of domestic violence perpetrated by their partners.

❖ In 1991, it was estimated that no more than twenty professionals in four American cities are adequately trained to deal effectively with lesbian and gay victims of violence.

These data suggest potential aging issues of abuse, domestic violence, lack of services, and lack of training of professionals. While these facts suggest that gay and lesbian Americans are a well-educated, high-income group, research is contradictory in gay gerontology.

Global View of Gay Men and Lesbians

Some countries have more tolerant legislation, others do not. More than three hundred lesbian and gay groups in fifty nations, working through Amnesty International and the International Lesbian and Gay Association, collect data on gay political prisoners and on sodomy laws. *Gay and Lesbian Stats: A Pocket Guide of Facts and Figures* publishes the following facts.

❖ Homosexual acts between consenting adults were no longer crimes in 1810 in France, 1917 in Russia, 1932 in Poland, 1942 in Switzerland, 1980 in Spain, and 1986 in New Zealand. Of 202 countries examined, some form of lesbian and gay movement exists in 56 countries. Lesbian- and gay-rights groups are in formation in 15 countries, but none are in 131 countries.

❖ A majority of the population favors equal rights for lesbians and gays in 11 countries, and a minority of the population favors equal rights for lesbians and gays in 47 countries.

❖ There is little public support of equal rights for lesbians and gays in 144 countries. Laws protect lesbians and gay men against discrimination in 6 countries.

❖ Of the 74 countries with laws prohibiting homosexual behavior, 72% are predominately Islamic countries, formerly communist, or previously part of the British Empire.

❖ In eight countries in which Islamic law applies, men who commit homosexual acts can be sentenced to death.

❖ In 23 of the 74 countries in which men can be punished for homosexual acts, women are not mentioned in the laws.

❖ The estimated number of gay men exterminated during the Third Reich ranges from 10,000 to 1,000,000.

❖ In Russia, 30% of the population is in favor of lesbian and gay rights; 33% is in favor of killing homosexuals.

❖ Before the dissolution of the Soviet Union, an average of 700 men were jailed each year for being gay.

❖ Since Lithuania gained its independence in 1990, 7 men have been sentenced to 3 to 8 years in prison for same-sex acts.

❖ In Austria, male and female homosexual acts were decriminalized in 1971, and homosexual prostitution was legalized in 1989.

❖ In a 1991 Gallup poll in Britain, 49% believed there were more gays now than there were 20 years ago, 53% considered homosexuality an acceptable "alternative life style," and 66% believed same-sex acts should be legal.

❖ Gay bashing in London rose 350% in 1989.

❖ The Congo Embassy in Brussels stated in 1987 that the "practice of homosexuality does not exist in the Congo."

❖ Sexual activity between adult males is illegal in South Africa.

❖ In 1993, the main political parties in South Africa endorsed a new constitution that includes forbidding discrimination based on sexual orientation.

❖ The Greater Johannesburg-Soweto lesbian and gay group, GLOW, founded in 1988, has nearly 400 members, 60% of whom are black.

❖ There have been targeted murders of lesbian and gay activists in Mexico.

❖ In Chile, lesbian and gay groups exist but are illegal. There is compulsory HIV testing of all gay men.

❖ The Japan International Lesbian and Gay Association, founded in 1984 with 2 members, now has 300 members. Of these, only 8 have announced publicly that they are homosexual.

❖ In China, being lesbian or gay is considered an illness and is treated with shock therapy or emetics.

❖ Tasmania is the only Australian state in which sexual acts between men are still illegal.

❖ In Sydney, Australia, 32% of non-domestic homicides in 1991 were anti-gay murders.

❖ In 1993, 55% of the Canadian population found homosexuality morally acceptable.

❖ In 1986, Denmark recognized lesbian and gay couples in inheritance-tax legislation.

❖ Denmark and Norway are the only two countries that allow lesbian and gay couples to marry.

❖ In the Netherlands, 90% of the population is in favor of equal rights for lesbians and gays.

(Singer and Deschamps 1994)

Being old and gay is a difficult challenge in a heterosexual society that discriminates against gay men and lesbians at all ages. In 1982, it was estimated that 3.5 million homosexual men and women older than 60 years were living in the United States. In 1992, estimates of the numbers of older gay men and lesbians ranged from 3% to 10% of the elderly population. Older gays and lesbians are disadvantaged in heterosexual society because of discrimination and in homosexual society due to ageism. In the 1970s, research on the gay population increased substantially (Kooden 1997).

Psychologically well-adjusted and self-accepting older gay men reportedly adapt well to the aging process (Kooden 1997). Research indicates that the gay male is even better off than his heterosexual counterpart because of past coping experiences. Earlier experiences in adapting to losses (of family or friends) may enable gay men and lesbians to function in later life with more flexibility. McDougall (1993) argues that older gay men and lesbians develop many strengths early in life that prepare them for old age such as cultivating non-career interests, increasing their personal autonomy, and preserving friendships outside of a lover relationship. A specific earlier coping mechanism is learning to live with the stigmatized identity of homosexuality. These strengths may better prepare the older homosexual to adjust to old age (McDougall 1993).

A study of gay males aging found no differences in unhappiness or depression as a function of age. Another study proposed that working through earlier life crises contributes to the strengths of older gay men. Studies of Australian homosexual males found that older gay men do not experience disengagement from the gay community and respondents expressed satisfaction with their homosexual lifestyle (Wahler and

Gabbay 1997). A study of Canadian gay men by Wahler and Gabbay found that factors of health, income, and education were predictive of satisfaction in late life.

Lesbian aging differs from the aging of non-lesbian women. The losses experienced by older women who lose a husband or heterosexual lover are not the same experiences for lesbians. The longer-lived heterosexual female will most likely not be able to replace a husband or male partner since men have shorter life expectancies. The lesbian most likely will remain with a partner; thus older lesbians are not lonely, isolated, and without anyone to love or care about them in old age (McDougall 1993).

Ethnic and Minority Lesbians and Gay Men

Research on lesbians and gay men is based on studies of white, middle-class respondents. Greene (1997) discusses ethnic minority lesbians and gay men within the framework of understanding the roles of men and women in ethnic cultures. While same-gender sexual behavior may not be uncommon, it is the overt acknowledgment and disclosure of a gay or lesbian identity that is likely to meet with disapproval in varying degrees across ethnic groups. For Latinos, women who label themselves as lesbians present a threat to the order of male dominance. Latino disapproval of homosexuality is more intense than the homophobia found in the Anglo community so that pressure to remain closeted is stronger. For a Latino, being gay or lesbian is an act of treason against the culture or the family (Greene 1997).

Asian Americans, Japanese, or Chinese are expected to marry, have children to carry on the family name, and maintain family responsibility for the elders. Open disclosure that one is gay or lesbian is a threat to the family line and a rejection of family responsibility (Greene 1997).

In African American families, gender roles are more flexible but homophobia among African Americans has multiple reasons. The strong presence of Christianity and the role of the church in the lives of African Americans reinforces homophobic attitudes (Greene 1997).

Native Americans have a cultural history of accepting and combining both male and female aspects of spirituality in behaviors and personality traits (Greene 1997).

Access to Services

Sexual orientation should not influence the ability of a client to receive help. Gay elderly people face many of the same problems of all elderly people as well as the prejudices of homophobia; these problems might include isolation, loneliness, and lack of access to help during illness. While the older person living in a community participates in community senior-center services and programs, gay men and lesbians do not become involved in local senior centers. In a negative environment, the older gay man or lesbian is not able to share problems of family and partners with others in a senior-center environment. Gay and lesbian older persons may not have support of family members or children during illness. Bereavement has a special impact on the gay and lesbian older person. The loss from death of a long-term partner is like the death of a marital partner, and the bereavement process is similar. However, the loss of a partner for a gay or lesbian person is not supported by society. Particular needs of older gay men and lesbians primarily are for more retirement communities and recreational activities; access to health care, long-term care, hospice; and recognition of elder-abuse problems in the gay community.

Access to health-care services is a significant problem for gay men and lesbians. While there are some age- and gender-specific services available, there are few services for the gay population. Nursing homes are not specifically focused on gay men and lesbians. Staff have little training in gerohomosexuality. Ageism is a problem in nursing homes and, in conjunction with homophobic attitudes, the gay older person is strongly disadvantaged (Hoctel 1999).

Psychotherapy focuses on homosexuality identity issues or the problems in relationships more than on issues of aging. Therapies lead to acceptance of alternative lifestyles for women. Feminist therapy and lesbian therapy is an affirmative therapy that has gained widespread popularity. Lesbians seek therapy for various reasons but among the most common are relationship problems, lesbian identity problems, and adjustment problems (Perkins 1997). Issues of aging and lesbianism are new research areas.

In most cities, gay men and lesbians have congregated in specific areas to live. There is an initiative in New York and San Francisco to develop retirement communities specifically for gay and lesbian older persons. An optimistic housing outlook for older gays and lesbians is developing. In the state of Washington there are plans for a twenty-two acre project that is similar to a development in Palmetto, Florida, and it is the first lesbian and gay retirement village in the United States (Hoctel 1999). In Amsterdam, assisted-living facilities exist that are primarily gay. Similar projects are being explored for San Francisco and Southern California. Prices for one project, Our Town, range from $200,000 to $400,000. Another project is Pod Cluster Housing Project in Michigan, built for seven women and including six to eight individual homes with a building in the center that connects to each home. Housing for gay men and lesbian elders is a growing need. Gay men and lesbians who live in rural areas have difficulty in finding housing that can fit their lifestyle.

Abuse of Lesbian and Gay Elders

Elder abuse of gay, lesbian, and transgender elders has not been extensively researched. Abuse in the gay population has been associated with homophobia in street violence and harassment, or in refusal of health professionals to provide care and services. Victims do not seek help because of risk of exposure. Legal discrimination makes it difficult for gay men or lesbians to leave abusive relationships because there are no legal ways to tap a partner's assets. Self-neglect is a serious problem. Internalized homophobia can lead to older persons accepting poor health and poor living conditions as being what they deserve. The current generation of lesbian and gay older persons has a history of hiding who they are and protecting their privacy. To allow someone into the home to provide personal care is seen as being a risk for exposure and chance of abuse or exploitation (Cook-Daniels 1997).

Advocacy Programs

SAGE (Seniors Active in a Gay Environment), a New York City agency established in 1977, provides access to professional medical and social services for older gay men and lesbians. SAGE provides social services, support programs, education, and advocacy for gay and lesbian seniors. The original mission of the organization was to provide care and support for homebound gay and lesbian seniors. SAGE chapters are in eleven American cities and one Canadian city (Kochman 1997).

The American Society on Aging's Lesbian and Gay Aging Issues Network (LGAIN) raises awareness of the special challenges facing older lesbians and gay men and the barriers encountered by this invisible segment of the population regarding housing, health care, long-term care, and social services. The network's goals include the following:

❖ To aid in dispelling stereotypes and myths about older lesbians and gay men.

❖ To encourage research that explores the experiences of older lesbians and gay men and documents their contributions and needs.

❖ To provide links between providers and agencies in health care, long-term care, and human services, creating greater awareness of the existence, needs, and lifestyles of older lesbians and gay men and promoting access to services.

❖ To work with lesbian and gay community organizations to create a greater awareness of the special gifts and talents of older lesbians and gay men and develop programs that respond to their needs. (American Society on Aging 1997)

Other advocacy organizations include The Society for Senior Gay and Lesbian Citizens/PROJECT RAINBOW in Los Angeles, The Gay and Lesbian Outreach to Elders in San Francisco, and Prime Timers in Boston. Gays and Lesbians Older and Wiser (GLOW) is a support group that is part of the services of a university-based geriatric clinic in Ann Arbor, Michigan. A resource guide published by the Lesbian and Gay Aging Association of San Francisco, California (1991), and provided by the National Association for Lesbian and Gay Gerontology, offers information on research, audiovisuals, and lists of organizations.

Older Women

"A new kind of society is evolving, and for the most part it is female."
Mylander quoted in Bonita 1993, 189

Generally women age better than do men; women live longer, eat healthier, avoid alcohol, develop social relationships, and have support networks to sustain themselves. Contemporary older women are healthier than their grandmothers, watch their weight, exercise more vigorously, seek medical attention more frequently, and are concerned about quality-of-life issues. But aging experiences for women are different from those faced by men. Women face physical, psychological, and social challenges in the aging process.

Physical Challenges

In 1991, the National Institute on Aging supported research that contributed to the knowledge of the epidemiology of diseases that affect women. Although women live longer than men, they suffer disproportionately from disability and chronic long-term illnesses. Disability threatens independence and contributes to high costs in health care. Disability in old age is associated with a poor quality of life, dependence on formal and informal caregivers, and substantial medical costs.

A particular age-related change for women is menopause, which is described as a physical event that occurs one year after the last menstrual period. There has been no documented similar time of life for men. In 1900, the average woman experienced menopause at about age 46 years. In 1999, the average age was 50 years. A woman can expect to live more than one-third of her life postmenopausal. ERT (estrogen replacement therapy) was introduced in the 1960s and is reported to be

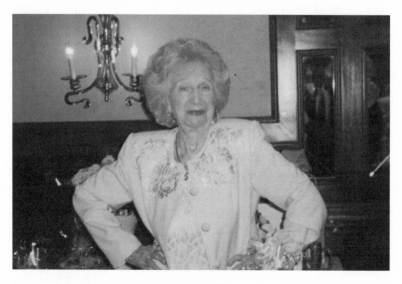

A woman can be proud of being 90 years old.

effective in reducing risks of heart disease and osteoporosis; research continues on its use as a potential risk for uterine cancer. ERT is recommended for the prevention of osteoporosis, a bone condition that affects more women than men. One of four white women older than 65 develops osteoporosis (National Institute on Aging 1997).

The National Institute on Aging (1997) recommends development of sufficient bone mass by regular exercise; calcium intake; and avoiding substances that interfere with bone metabolism such as coffee, smoking, and red meat. Bone maturity reaches its peak at about age 35 years. Bone loss occurs with age. ERT is recommended for persons who have close relatives (mother or sister) who have osteoporosis; those who are fair-skinned, slim, or heavy smokers; or those who have taken bone-robbing drugs such as cortisone drugs for other diseases.

Osteoarthritis is a physical threat for older women. Women are one and one-half times more likely than men to develop osteoarthritis, which affects any joint in the back, knees, hips, and neck. The symptoms respond to anti-inflammatory drugs and exercises. It is a chronic disease that is disabling. (See Appendix B for a self-administered bone test.)

Heart disease is not primarily a disease that affects men. After menopause, women lose the cardiovascular protection of estrogen and they are at risk of dying of heart disease. Between ages 45 and 54 years, women die of cardiovascular disease at the rate of 84 per 100,000 per year. For those older than age 65, the rate reaches 1,958 per 100,000 per year, which is almost as high as the rate for men that age. One of four women older than 65 years has a cardiovascular disease such as coronary heart disease, hypertension, angina, and stroke. Women develop cardiovascular disease an average of ten to twenty years later than men do even though they have the same risk factors of smoking, blood cholesterol levels, and family histories of heart disease (National Institute on Aging 1997). Although women develop milder forms of heart disease, when a woman does develop severe heart disease she is more likely to have serious consequences. A woman is more likely than a man to suffer a second heart attack within five years of the first, and is less likely to benefit from aspirin as a blood thinner to prevent heart attacks. She is less likely to benefit from bypass surgery.

A woman's risk of hypertension is greater than a man's with advancing age. After the age of 65, higher proportions of women than men have problems with blood pressure. Women are more likely than men to have elevated levels of cholesterol. High cholesterol levels are associated with cardiovascular disease and are caused by an inherited tendency to accumulate blood fats, a diet high in fats and cholesterol, or a combination of the two. Nearly one-half of women older than age 55 have high blood cholesterol, compared to less than one-third of men the same age.

Older women are particularly at risk of death from cancer. One of eight deaths in women older than 65 years is due to cancer, particularly cancer of the digestive organs (such as the colon), the breast, and the lungs. Breast cancer is the most common. One in ten women will develop breast cancer in her lifetime. Another widespread problem for older women is urinary incontinence. Stress incontinence is frequent in older women because the pelvic floor muscles tend to become weaker with age after childbirth and in women who are overweight.

Psychological Challenges

Alzheimer's disease affects more women than men primarily because it is a disease that generally affects those older than 80 years. Women in their eighties outnumber men by at least two to one. Older women have higher rates of depression and they are twice as likely as men, at any age, to become depressed. Older women are at greater risk for misdiagnosis and lack of treatment in spite of the fact that depression in late life significantly improves after treatment. Women show a decline in rates of suicide as they age, with the peak period at age 54 when 10 per 100,000 commit suicide (National Institute on Aging 1997). While some women may find themselves without a husband or children to care for and at risk of depression, others have resilient coping skills and tend to maintain their social ties and support networks.

A particularly important psychological problem for older women is low self-esteem in a society that values youth and beauty. Women experience the negative effects of being old in a society that values sex appeal, the ability to bear children, and youth. Age compounds a woman's already devalued status.

Women suffer psychological damage, particularly in divorce, and especially by husbands who value younger women. Women tend to incorporate their physical image into their psychological image and suffer a loss of self-esteem as they age and no longer have the same physical appearance of youth. Older women face a challenge aging in a society that does not value older women.

A familiar story is of the husband who divorces his wife of twenty-five or thirty years; she changed physically and no longer has the "beauty" she had when she was 20 or 30 years old. He divorces his wife (age 50 to 60) and marries a younger woman. Bonita (1993, 192) states, "Beauty does not stand up well to age." The increase in late-life divorces perpetuates this age-old trend of the older man wanting a younger woman. While the bodily changes occur in both men and women, women tend to be more humiliated by the changes.

Social Challenges

Social challenges for women include economic disadvantages. Women older than 65 years account for more than 70% of the poor population (Hooyman and Kiyak 1996). Nearly 15% of women live in poverty, compared to 8% of men. The median income of older women is 58% less than that of older men. Unmarried women living alone and ethnic women are more likely to be poor. About 66% of older African American women are not living with family, and 61% of Hispanic women live alone and have incomes below the poverty level. Differences in employment history, types of work, earnings, and lack of pensions account for the high rates of older women who are poor.

In 1950, the labor force participation of women was 9.7%. Women in the present cohort of those older than 65 years did not have long-term careers, worked part-time if at all, and have little or no retirement incomes. The primary source of income for women older than 65 years in 1989 was Social Security. Women are primarily dependent upon men for their income and their retirement benefits. A serious problem resulting from this dependency is that divorced and widowed women are at risk for poverty because their income is dependent upon a deceased husband's retirement income, which may not exist after his death.

Divorced older women are at greater risk of poverty. Sixteen percent of divorces affect women age 45 and older (Hooyman and Kiyak 1996). Older divorced women are particularly at risk since Social Security regulations do not provide payments for marriages of less than ten years. A divorced spouse who has been married for at least ten years is entitled to 50% of the former spouse's benefits. Traditionally, women who have interrupted careers to leave the labor force for child rearing are less likely to have private pensions.

The future for women remains unclear. Economically, women encounter glass-ceiling barriers in the workforce. Women are more likely to have part-time jobs and poorly paid jobs in service industries.

Older women have limited opportunities to remarry due to the higher proportion of women who survive to old age than men. At age 65, remarriage rates are 2 per 1,000 for women compared to 17 per 1,000 for men (Hooyman and Kiyak 1996). The chances of remarriage decline with age. The widow faces psychological and social challenges. Ruth, who was married to Morris for 40 years, writes:

> It is exactly four months since my husband passed away. Most of our conversations while he was ill were of the wonderful times we had together. My children and grandchildren would like to see me continue with my life but it is so hard without Morris by my side.

Older Women in Other Countries

Women outlive men in all countries. Women's greater longevity and pattern of marrying older men create substantially higher proportions of women who live alone. Older women are more likely to be poorer in old age than men for various reasons such as involvement in child rearing, interruption of careers for child-care responsibilities, less investment in training and education, labor-force discrimination, low-paying jobs, and, in some countries, ineligibility for spouse's pension or land inheritance. Of the estimated 1.3 billion people living in poverty, more than 70% are older women (UNDPI 1996).

Women face more of the burdens of caregiving for older parents. Adult daughters are the primary caregivers of aging parents. Adult daughters, in their sixties and seventies, provide care for parents in their eighties and nineties. Women who never married or who do not have children are at greater risk for institutionalization for social rather than medical reasons. More than 70% of nursing home patients are women and the majority have never married or are widowed. One in four women older than 85 years who are in nursing homes are widowed or were never married (Hooyman and Kiyak 1996).

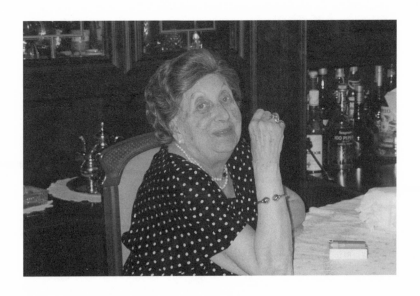

Women of today, both in Sicily and around the world, can face widowhood with greater optimism than did women of yesterday.

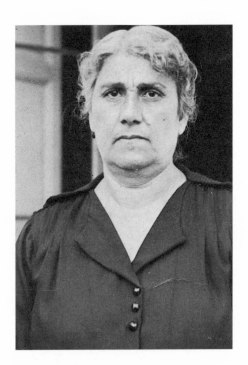

The support systems women develop throughout their lives serve to reward them with the social resources and intimate relationships that positively affect quality of life as they age. Women's roles as unpaid caregivers for children and older persons are devalued and often have negative effects on health and economic status. The woman of the 1990s can be described as a superwoman, balancing career, child-care, and family responsibilities with social and economic responsibilities.

Ageism and sexism are found in most countries in the world. Bonita (1993, 190) states that ageism and sexism have been termed the "twin prejudices." In New Zealand in 1991, there were 214,000 women older than 65 years, which was 12.5% of all women and 6.3% of the total population. There were approximately 155,000 men older than 65 years, which was 9% of all men and 4.6% of the total population. In New Zealand, there are 138 older women for every 100 older men, a difference referred to as the feminization of old age or the gender gap.

Women live an average of 77 years, or six years longer than men do. Women live longer than men for a variety of reasons including environmental issues, health habits, and social or cultural habits such as smoking or alcohol use. In a New Zealand Survey, 60% of older women had never smoked cigarettes, compared with 21% of older men. New Zealand women are more interested in healthy aging and positive self-care, are more likely to report illness, and place a greater reliance on medical care for their well-being. For every widower in New Zealand there are five widows. A woman who loses her husband can expect to live about 18 years, on average, as a widow. One in three marriages ends in divorce and 7% of divorced women do not choose to remarry; therefore, more women will live alone or with other people. In a study of residents and patients in a New Zealand long-term care facility, 44% of women lived in long-term care facilities compared with only 22% of men. Another New Zealand study showed that women in institutions were at greater risk of erosion of their independence due to paternalistic attitudes toward older persons (Bonita 1993).

In Korea, the population of older adults older than 65 years constituted 6.8% of the population in 2000. The average life expectancy is 74.3 years. Life expectancy for women is 77.3 years and for men it is 71.3 years, a difference of six years (Yoon 1995). Studies of the changing relationships of older Koreans in the family indicate increasing conflicts between mother-in-law and daughter-in-law. In Korean society, sons are responsible for care of aging mothers (filial responsibility). The aging woman with no son is considered a burden to society.

Under the Confucian system, the father is the head of the household, and the social status of women is very low but maternal status is highly valued. When a man ages, he hands over all of his property to his son, and the aged wife hands over her household management rights to her daughter-in-law. The aged family enjoys the respect of the next generation. Women in Korea outlive their husbands and tend to marry younger men. Of married women age 60 and older in 1992, 34.5% had a spouse and 65.5% were widowed. In addition, the older man is three times more likely than the older woman to remarry. A new experience for Korean families is having time alone after the children are married. Korean older women, as in most underdeveloped countries, are discriminated against economically and socially (Yoon 1995).

The Future of Older Women

The future of older women globally is positive in developed countries and changing for the better in underdeveloped countries. Younger women in Islamic countries, such as Afghanistan, suffer discrimination and abuse. In India, female children are aborted. In China, female children are most often unwanted, even for adoptions. In underdeveloped countries, women are paid the lowest wages and work in deplorable conditions.

In Western and Eastern countries, women are breaking the glass ceiling and accomplishing unexpected goals. Women are visible in political situations and economic arenas. Women all over the world seek youth and beauty. Women of the baby boomer generation will change the image of beauty around the world by maintaining an agelessness as long as possible. Ageism in the work place, in the media, and in everyday life is challenged by modern women. Women face physical, psychological, and social challenges in the future with resilience.

Ethnic and Minority Older Adults

In America and in other countries of the world, ethnic and minority persons experience aging with more difficulties than does the majority population. Access to health and social services, differences in cultural norms of immigrant groups, language problems, lack of appreciation for cultural beliefs and values, and a lack of culturally sensitive programs and services are problems for ethnic and minority older persons. In the United States, disadvantaged minorities die younger and have more illnesses (hypertension, diabetes, AIDS, accidents, alcoholism). Minority women experience more illnesses than do white women and have lower rates of life expectancy. An inverse relationship exists between economic status and mortality, morbidity, and the inequality of physical health between whites and ethnic minority populations (Markides and Black 1996).

In the United States, the non-Hispanic white proportion of the population is expected to decrease from 74% in 1995, to 72% in 2000, and to 64% in 2020. The African American population is expected to double its 1995 size to 61 million by the middle of this century. The highest rates of increase will be in the Hispanic, Asian, and Pacific Islander populations. The Hispanic population is predicted to be the second-largest racial/ethnic group, following the non-Hispanic white population (Mui, Choi, and Monk 1998). Ethnicity is defined by Holzberg as:

> Social differentiation based on such cultural criteria as a sense of peoplehood, shared history, a common place of origin, language, dress and free preferences, and participation in particular clubs or voluntary associations, engenders a sense of exclusiveness and self-awareness that one is a member of a distinct and bounded social group. But it is not the ethnic content per se that constitutes the diacritic of social differentiation. More important for the purposes of social distance are the feelings of shared particularity, self-identification, and membership in ethnic exclusive associations. (1982, 252)

Ethnic groups share positive traits within cultures: the support of cultural norms, family traditions, and a sense of peoplehood. However, there are negative aspects of immigration and lack of acculturation, most significantly language difficulties and changes in cultural expectations.

Mui, Choi, and Monk (1998) researched white (non-Hispanic), African American, and Hispanic elders in terms of psychological well-being and depressive symptoms, life strain, and coping resources. Hispanic frail elders reported the highest mean scores of depressive symptoms, and African Americans reported the lowest mean scores. Among Mexican Americans, Puerto Ricans, and Cuban American elders, Cuban American elders were healthier and financially better off than members of the other two groups.

In a study of nursing home admissions, white frail elders were 73% more likely than African American and Hispanic elders to apply for nursing home admission. Predictors were advanced age, cognitive and functional impairments, low income, number of formal services used, living alone, and number of unmet needs. The availability of informal support was not a significant factor. The use of community and home-based services by African Americans, Hispanics, and white frail elders is low for all three groups. The likelihood that elders will use services such as Meals on Wheels was positively associated with ability to read English. In terms of caregiver support, the three racial/ethnic groups were not significantly different in the size of their caregiver networks. Whites and Hispanics rely mostly on immediate family while African Americans rely on a network of friends and neighbors. African American caregivers reported low levels of stress. White and Hispanic caregivers reported high levels of stress. Hispanics used the least number of formal services. While minority elderly are disadvantaged in income and health, there is no evidence that psychological well-being is at risk. Psychological well-being decreases once health, income, and marital status are controlled.

Markides and Black (1996) argue that few psychiatric epidemiological studies include large numbers of ethnic elderly. Increases in longevity patterns of ethnic minority are expected in the general population. Greater use of nursing homes and long-term care by ethnic minority elderly is also expected since caregiving women compromise their own future economic security to care for family members. Drug abuse and AIDS disproportionately affect minority groups and increase the dependence of younger persons on middle-aged and older persons for support.

Ethnic and minority groups are found in New Zealand (the Maori), in Australia (the Aboriginal and Torres Strait Islander peoples), and in many European countries in which ethnic groups have migrated. In most countries, ethnic older adults are disadvantaged in health care, social situations, and financial situations. While minority and ethnic elderly are economically and socially disadvantaged, the increasing numbers of elderly in these groups will demand changes. The experience of aging will differ for the next cohort of older persons.

Summary

There is controversy in gay gerontology about the successful aging of older gay men and lesbians. Studies indicate that the older gay and lesbian person faces loneliness, isolation, sexlessness, poor psychological adjustment, anxiety, sadness and depression, sexual predation on the gay youth, and ageism from a youthful gay culture. Contrary to these findings are studies that report that older gay men and lesbians are less worried about exposure of homosexuality with increasing age, are not lonely, are more self-accepting, have a better self-concept than younger gays and lesbians, and deal with aging more positively because of having adapted to a stigmatized identity earlier in life. More research on gay gerontology is necessary as well as education and training in gerohomosexuality for health professionals.

The future for women is promising even though current situations are challenging. In Western and Eastern countries, women are accomplishing unexpected goals in political situations and economic arenas. Baby boomer women will attempt to maintain an agelessness as long as possible. Ageism in the work place, in the media, and in everyday life is challenged by modern women as they face physical, psychological, and social challenges in the future with resilience.

Increases in longevity patterns of ethnic minority are predictable in the general population. Ethnic and minority older adults are anticipated to increase in numbers and need improved health and social services. The experiences of aging for women, gay men and lesbians, and ethnic and minority groups will challenge social and political systems.

References

American Society on Aging. 1997. *Lesbian and Gay Aging Issues Network (LGAIN)*. American Society on Aging. On-line: http://www.asaging.org/networks/lgain/outward.htn.

Bonita, Ruth. 1993. Older women: A growing force. In *New Zealand's aging society: The implications,* edited by Peggy Koopman-Boyden. Wellington, New Zealand: Daphne Brasell Associates Press.

Cook-Daniels, Loree. 1997. *Outword: Abuse of lesbian, gay, and transgender elders.* American Society on Aging. On-line: http://www.asaging.org/networks/lgain/outward.htn.

Greene, Beverly. 1997. Ethnic minority lesbians and gay men: Mental health and treatment issues. In Vol. 3 of *Ethnic and cultural diversity among lesbians and gay men,* edited by Beverly Greene. Thousand Oaks, Calif.: Sage Publications.

Hoctel, Patrick D. 1999. Optimistic housing outlook for older gays, lesbians. *Aging Today* (Sept./Oct.): 7.

Holzberg, C. 1982. Ethnicity and aging: Anthropological perspectives on more than just minority elderly. *Gerontologist* 22: 249–57.

Hooyman, N., and H. A. Kiyak. 1996. *Social gerontology: A multidisciplinary perspective.* 4th ed. Boston: Allyn and Bacon.

Kochman, Arlene. 1997. Gay and lesbian elderly: Historical overview and implications for social work practice. *Journal of Gay and Lesbian Social Services* 6 (1): 1–9.

Kooden, Harold. 1997. Successful aging in the middle-aged gay man: A contribution to developmental theory. *Journal of Gay and Lesbian Social Services* 6 (3): 21–42.

Markides, K. S., and S. A. Black. 1996. Race, ethnicity, and aging: The impact of inequality. In *Handbook of aging and the social sciences,* edited by R. H. Binstock and L. K. George. 4th ed. San Diego, Calif.: Academic Press.

McDougall, G. J. 1993. Therapeutic issues with gay and lesbian elders. *Clinical Gerontologist* 14 (1): 45–57.

Mui, A. C., N. G. Choi, and A. Monk. 1998. *Long-term care and ethnicity.* Westport, Conn.: Auburn House.

National Institute on Aging. 1997. *Answers about: The aging woman and man.* U.S. Department of Health and Human Services, Public Health Service, and National Institutes of Health.

Perkins, Rachel. 1997. Therapy for lesbians? The case against. In *Classics in lesbian studies,* edited by Esther D. Rothblum. Binghamton, N.Y.: Haworth Press.

Singer, B. L., and D. Deschamps. 1994. *Gay and lesbian stats: A pocket guide of facts and figures.* New York: The New Press.

United Nations Department of Public Information (UNDPI). 1996. *International Year of Older Persons: The aging of the world's population.*

respite from caregiving responsibilities, but respite programs are being developed to help family members with caregiving. Home health-care services are quite extensive in some countries (such as Australia), fledgling in North America, and almost nonexistent in Asian countries. Social services are provided by senior centers and religious organizations. Programs that protect from abuse and exploitation differ in each country.

Recreation and leisure enhance quality of life. Older persons are involved in traveling, sports, computer use, and many non-traditional activities such as skydiving and scuba diving. Senior centers are common places for recreational activities in America, and family centers serve the same function in Europe, Asia, Australia, and New Zealand. Protection and advocacy programs for older adults offer help in dealing with elder abuse and legal issues. Educational programs for older persons include the possibility of returning to school, education for recreation, and Elderhostel. Finally, intergenerational programs continue to explore how the old and young can help each other.

Publicly Supported Programs and Services

In Australia, New Zealand, Europe, Canada, and Asia, universal coverage for health programs is widespread; however, publicly supported income programs vary. Underdeveloped countries may provide public income-support for poor persons. Governments are re-examining current systems or developing new pension plans for retirement. In the United States, Social Security is a federal income support program based on employee contributions. Medicare, begun in 1965 under the Social Security Act, is a national health-insurance program for those persons who contributed to the program as employees. Both programs are currently under scrutiny.

Australia provides publically funded pensions to older persons. In addition to the public pension, Australia has a compulsory Superannuation System, which facilitates the accumulation of private savings for retirement. The Superannuation Guarantee legislation requires employers to provide a minimum level of Superannuation support for employees who earn $450 or more per month or become liable to pay a Supernannuation Guarantee Charge. In 1997–1998, employers were required to make contributions equivalent to 6% of an employee's earnings, a figure that will rise to 9% by 2003. As a result, Australians are expected to have a much higher retirement income in the future than they would have with an age pension.

The Australian age pension was introduced in 1909 to provide a safety net for older people who are unable to provide for themselves financially. As of 1997, the rate was $347 a fortnight for a single person and $290 for each member of a married couple. The Australian age pension is a flat-rate, non-contributory payment funded from general revenue and not linked to previous labor-force participation. It is income- and asset-tested and is intended for the financially needy. The age pension is payable to men starting at age 65 years and to women starting at age 61 years. With the increasing numbers of older persons, Australians are encouraged to save for retirement. Publicly supported pensions are unstable in countries such as Chile, Argentina, the United States, and Germany.

Health Care Programs and Services

In the United States, Medicare, a national health insurance for older persons, is linked to Social Security payments. Those persons who are eligible for Social Security payments are eligible for Medicare coverage. This health insurance covers adults older than 65 years who contributed to the Social Security System, those who are entitled to Social Security disability payments for twenty-four months or more, and those persons with end-stage kidney disease.

Medicare insurance is divided into two parts, part A and part B. Part A is funded by employee and employer contributions. Each pays 1.45% of payroll, and self-employed persons pay 2.9%. Part B is funded by monthly premiums paid by the beneficiaries and general-fund revenues. Premiums cover about 36% of the costs and federal funds cover the remainder. All persons who are eligible for Social Security benefits or Railroad Retirement benefits are eligible. There is no cost for part A, but those who participate in part B pay a monthly premium ($43.80 in 1997) and $100 per year deductible for physician services.

Part A covers costs associated with hospitalization and some post-hospitalization, skilled-nursing facility care, home health care, hospice care, and blood transfusions. Part A pays for hospital services (90 days per benefit period), skilled-nursing care (100 days following a 3-day hospital stay), some home health care services, and hospice care. Part B pays for the costs of physician services, outpatient hospital services, medical equipment and supplies, some rehabilitation services, blood tests, urinalyses, blood, and some ambulatory surgical services. Older adults can supplement Medicare insurance by purchasing Medigap insurance policies, which are designed to pay deductible, co-payments, and the remaining 20% of the charges for physicians and hospitals that Medicare does not pay.

Medicaid provides medical assistance for low-income families and individuals, and state and federal governments jointly fund the program. It is a means-tested program. Each state develops its own range of services and eligibility requirements. Medicaid programs vary from state to state. Because each state determines eligibility guidelines, the state also determines coverage. Basic services include inpatient and outpatient hospital services, physician services, nursing home services, health clinics, home health care, laboratory and X-rays, dental services, drugs, optometrist services, and prosthetic devices. States can require beneficiaries to enroll in managed-care plans. Delaware, Florida, Hawaii, Illinois, Kentucky, Maryland, Massachusetts, Ohio, Oklahoma, Oregon, Rhode Island, Tennessee, and Vermont established an all-managed-care Medicaid program (Wacker, Roberto, and Piper 1998).

Managed-care programs (HMOs) in the United States have proliferated to control rising costs of health care. Managed care is defined as the effort to coordinate, rationalize, and channel the use of services to achieve desired access, service, and outcomes while controlling costs (Wacker, Roberto, and Piper 1998). HMOs provide managed care that includes comprehensive health services at a fixed cost. Controversy exists concerning the advantages and disadvantages of managed care and HMO programs. Advantages include having available a wide range of services at a small charge or co-payment. Disadvantages include restrictions of services and physicians and denial of services by insurance companies.

While Australians older than 65 years make up 12% of the country's total population, they spent 35% of the $31 billion in total expenditures for health services in 1993–1994. Health expenditures for persons older than 65 years were 3.8 times higher than for those younger than 65 years. In Australia, one type of program is the brokerage-type for home-based-care community packages in which a person can purchase services as needed with government funding. Germany instituted a lump-sum payment for caregivers with restrictions that services will not be purchased in public programs and health-care costs must not include nursing homes. Long-term care, whether home-based or institutional, such as nursing homes, is an essential component of health-care services for older persons.

Nursing Homes

Case Example—The Nursing Home

Catherine T, age 90 years, had been living in an apartment in Brooklyn, New York, for more than 50 years. She has five children—two sons and three daughters. Her three daughters live nearby and visit every day. During the day, a home-health aide came to shop for her, wash clothes, clean the apartment, and help her shower. In the past year, she has become frail and tires easily. She suffers from shortness of breath (heart disease), diabetes, kidney disease, and hypertension. Mrs. T was no longer able to leave the house without assistance. She was fearful of being alone in the evenings and suffered panic attacks. She and her daughters arranged for nursing home placement. Initially, she felt safe and well cared for with a large staff of nurses and physicians. She attended physical therapy sessions daily to strengthen her leg muscles. However, within a few weeks of entering the nursing home she became depressed. The majority of patients in the facility had dementia and her sources of socialization were limited to her daughters' daily visits. She found that staff complained of being overworked and understaffed. She is attended to based on the staff's schedule and not on her needs. She regrets her decision to move each day.

The quality and costs of nursing homes has been studied extensively over the last two decades. The 1996 Medical Expenditure Survey in the Nursing Home Component reports the high costs to the federal and state budgets for nursing home care. Nursing homes are heavily regulated to protect patients from emotional, physical, and financial abuses. However, nursing home abuses are still rampant. The failure of long-term settings to attend to problems in mental health is a pervasive problem (Cohen 1997).

Older adults fear losing their independence because loss of independence usually leads to nursing home placement. Although many nursing homes maintain quality standards, the lack of concern for individualization of patient care perpetuates a fear of living in a setting that claims to be home but is a medical facility. The term "nursing home" is an oxymoron. Nursing homes are medical facilities that infrequently resemble homes even if the furnishings are home-like. The routines of care, the concern for regulatory procedures, and the lack of individualization in food and services are institutional and not home-like, despite claims of being a home.

In Western Pennsylvania, a facility for patients with Alzheimer's disease was designed to provide a setting that seems like a home. It is small, intimate, and personal. The facility has three houses linked to a main building, with each house surrounded by a picket fence. In each unit, twelve residents each have private rooms and private bathrooms. Each unit has a kitchen, and a staff member serves meals around the clock to meet the individual demands of Alzheimer's patients. Circular walkways permit the residents to wander freely. Evaluation has shown that these residents have slower rates of deterioration than those being cared for in conventional nursing homes, and the operational costs are reported to be 20% lower than traditional nursing homes (Does the care suit the client? 1997). Unfortunately, this type of facility is unusual.

Hospice Care

Case Example—Hospice Care

Myra's father, David S, is terminally ill and lives in Florida, while she lives in Texas. She is his only child. Mr. S lives in a senior apartment complex and had friends provide some help with his meals. He hired a part-time housekeeper to help with housecleaning and shopping. In the advanced stages of cancer, he is physically weak and deteriorating. Myra talked to him about hospice care. Both she and her father have little information about hospice services and many misconceptions about the care he can receive from a hospice program.

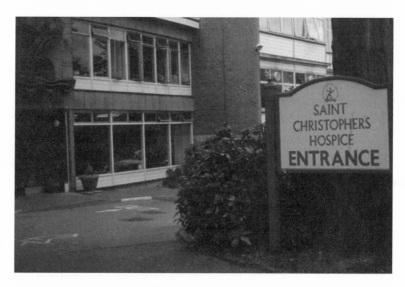

St. Christopher's Hospice, London, was the first facility of its kind.

Hospice began in the Middle Ages when monks cared for people dying in the streets. In England, St. Christopher's Hospice was founded in 1967 by Dame Cicely Saunders; it is the model for today's hospice. Hospice care is based on these principles, which have withstood time and cultures.

❖ There should be skilled analysis of pain and symptom control.

❖ Input from a multidisciplinary team is needed to relieve the experience of pain and enable a person to face what is happening in his or her individual way.

❖ Pain relief should be available whether the person is at home, hospice, or hospital, in space freed from the presence or threat of pain, breathlessness, and other forms of suffering.

❖ An important goal is maximizing the potential remaining to a patient or family, not only in quality of physical ease but also in relationships.

❖ The whole family, whatever its nature, is the focus and unit of care both during and after the patient's illness and in bereavement.

❖ Helping the dying is a taxing task for a single person. (Saunders 1997) addition, only 13.9% stated that they wanted to live with their children when they were older.

Attitudes are changing and the tradition of children supporting their elderly parents is disappearing. There are free homes for the poor aged and free nursing homes for anyone who needs placement. Private homes and private nursing homes for the aged are being developed. In 1960, there were 2,314 residents in institutional facilities for the aged; by 1993, this number had grown to 7,525 residents. Although this number is still a small proportion of the total population of 41 million, institutional residences are increasing. Korea has a housing shortage. Housing prices in Korea increase at higher rates than do consumer prices. Land is scarce. The government is encouraging the building of *silver towns*, which are privately owned homes for the aged with medical care available for the residents. More than 74.5% of those older than 45 years of age prefer to live in retirement communities rather than with their children. Korea is at the beginning stages of housing development for its elderly population (Kim 1997).

In India, the elderly prefer to live with their children. Sons are responsible for the care of their parents. In 1991, India's population was 844 million persons. In 2000, the elderly population was 75.9 million. India has more elderly people than the total population of many countries including Iran, Egypt, Turkey, Thailand, Ethiopia, Germany, and France. In India, the majority of the population lives in rural areas and the family provides physical, social, and economic support for the aged. The care of elderly parents is based on mutual exchange over a lifetime. While the majority of older persons live with their children, 12,758,610 persons, or 30%, have no families to live with or cannot live with their families. For this group, old-age homes are needed. Most old-age homes are public charities. The existing number of homes available is not sufficient to meet the needs of older persons who need care (Kara 1997).

Denmark has changed its housing policies in the past fifteen years. Nursing homes are no longer being built. Staying in the home is the goal, with support coming in the form of home nursing care, which is given to everyone free of charge and according to need. Fifteen percent of the population is older than 65 years of age, or 793,000 individuals of a population of 5,213,000 persons. Families are relatively small.

Most elderly people live alone. There is little potential for informal care from daughters because most are in the labor market. Only 7% of the elderly live in institutions. Elderly Danes have economic resources and want to live an independent and secure life in retirement (Lindstrom 1997).

Japan's older population is increasing at a phenomenal rate and the country is facing a housing problem. In 2020, more than 30% of the population will be older than 65 years and the birth rate, which was 1.43 in 1995, is declining. In 1969, paired apartments were constructed to enable elderly persons to live next door to their children. In 1975, large apartments were permitted to enable parents and children to live together. Children are moving to large cities, while elderly persons tend to prefer to live independently in their neighborhoods. While policy over the last forty years encouraged more housing for aged persons, another plan is building a barrier-free independent-living environment that can be used for a lifetime (Kose 1997).

Social Support Programs and Services

Case Example—The Senior Center

The Capital Senior Center has a membership of 3,000 seniors older than age 55. Each day, meals are served and exercise and yoga programs are available. Bill T, age 73 years, has been actively involved in the Center's activities since its opening in 1997. The majority of daily participants are older women. Hot lunch is offered at a cost of $3.00. Transportation is available. A swimming pool and an exercise room are on the premises. Special events are planned such as educational lectures, holiday parties, and day or weekend trips.

Senior centers are the focus for community social activities for older Americans. Family centers serve the same function in Europe, Asia, Australia, and New Zealand. According to the National Institute of Senior Centers, senior centers are based on the philosophy that

Aging is a normal developmental process; that human beings need peers with whom they can interact and who are available as a source of encouragement and support; and that adults have the right to have a voice in determining matters in which they have a vital interest. As such, the center is a major community institution that is geared to maintain good mental health and to prevent breakdown and deterioration of mental, emotional and social functioning of the older person. (Wacker, Roberto, and Piper 1998, 115)

In the United States, senior centers were created in 1965 with the passage of the Older Americans Act (OAA). In 1973, the OAA mandated that, with a new Title V program, senior centers must provide nutritional services and these sites are known as congregate meal sites, or they deliver meals to the home as Meals on Wheels programs. Multipurpose senior centers deliver a range of services. Between 5 and 8 million older adults attend senior centers (Krout 1998). The participants are usually female and live alone or with a non-relative.

About twenty years ago, senior center participants were in their sixties. The average age of participants is now in the eighties. A younger cohort of older adults is not participating in senior center activities. Older adults of color are less likely to attend senior centers. A national sample of recreation and senior center directors estimated the percentage of their participants by ethnic group and reported that older African Americans made up 8% of the participants; older Hispanics, 5%; and older Asian and Native Americans, 2% (Wacker, Roberto, and Piper 1998). But some centers reach out to specific groups. The Gay and Lesbian Outreach to Elders Senior Center (GLOE) is a senior center for gay men and lesbians. In some ethnic areas such as San Francisco, New York, and New Mexico, senior center participants are primarily Chinese, Japanese, African American, or Native American.

Programs offered at senior centers vary from community services, to group and individual programs. These programs include recreational programs, health and mental health programs, educational programs, nutritional and educational programs, travel programs, arts and music programs, employment programs, intergenerational programs, information and referral services, support groups and counseling, social action, volunteer opportunities, fitness programs, blood-pressure checks, vision screening tests, adult day care, legal assistance, and even financial educational programs. Senior centers attract the healthy elderly in their seventies and eighties. An Internet source providing links to state and area agencies that can help identify local services for seniors is Eldercare Locator at http://www.eldercare.gov

Case Example—The Religious Organization

Dr. K, a professor at the local university, is a volunteer in the Korean church in his community. On Saturday, he offers seminars on health issues, depression, anxiety, cultural conflicts, and family issues. His wife, Eunice, a nurse, provides blood-pressure checks, and medication monitoring; she also teaches seminars on diabetes, high blood pressure, and similar topics. Mr. L, a pharmacist, offers medication checks. Mr. K, a businessperson, offers business advice for new entrepreneurs. Mr. S, a lawyer, discusses legal options, and Mrs. S, a teacher, provides English lessons. The Korean church congregation provides lunch and transportation.

Religious organizations provide a variety of support programs for older adults such as transportation, travel support groups, educational programs, and social services. Brashears and Roberts (1996) report on an innovative social-service program of the Second Baptist Church in Kansas City, Missouri. The Second Baptist Church is the oldest African American Baptist church in Kansas City, with a congregation of 700 members. In 1987, a social worker was added to the church staff in a paid position. The social worker provides direct services to the members of the church and their families, and serves as the program administrator in the church's organizational structure. The social worker provides case management; support services to the homebound and institutionalized members; support services to members and families experiencing distress, health crises, and terminal illness; family counseling services; and referrals for emergency community services (Brashears and Roberts 1996).

Churches and synagogues offer a variety of programs for older persons, from medical assistance to financial assistance. The Brookland Baptist Church in West Columbia, South Carolina, maintains a credit union for its members. Religious organizations maintain nursing homes and housing for older persons, as well as day-care programs. However, the churches can do more to fill the gap that governments, worldwide, are not able to manage. The spirit of collaboration between church and government must be renewed to meet the needs of older persons in each community (Tirrito and Spencer-Amado, 2000).

Intergenerational Programs and Services

Case Example—Intergenerational Programs

In Seoul, Korea, family centers incorporate children's day-care programs with teenage sports, tutoring, parenting-skills programs, and elder-care programs (exercise, social activities, and recreation). On a typical day, a parent brings the children to day care and the mother-in-law to senior care. After a day at work, the parent comes to the center to pick up the teenage children, young children, and mother-in-law. Each of those at the family center has been involved in various activities separately and, sometimes, intergenerationally.

At the Australian Catholic University, students attending classes bring their young children to the day-care center, where teenagers and older persons in the community provide day care without charge.

In England at St. Christopher's Hospice, a free community day-care center for neighborhood children offers the terminally ill an opportunity to interact with young children and offers parents free day care.

Intergenerational programs explore how the old and young can help each other. In one high school program, students are linked to homebound elderly; in another program in New York City, seniors who speak foreign languages are linked with students and help them improve their ability to speak and understand a foreign language. Linking students with hospitals and nursing homes helps students to learn about various health professions.

Younger children often participate in singing groups in nursing homes or senior housing developments. Church groups link young and old together in church-related study programs. Senior centers link students with seniors in computer work. Working with computers removes language barriers. Day-care programs for adults and day care for children are reciprocal arrangements of care. In Korea, the family center is a place where intergenerational programming occurs spontaneously. Children, adults, adolescents, and older persons come together in an exchange of services. Adults take care of young children, and young people help older people. Old people and younger people are interdependent, and programs need to build on reciprocity.

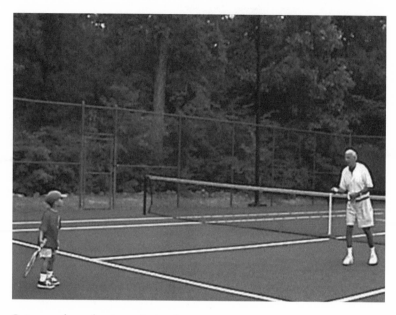

Being together enhances understanding.

Summary

Programs and services for older adults are diverse globally. A brief description of these programs gives the reader an opportunity to know what is available and to explore references or web sites for in-depth information about these programs. From the Internet it is possible to access information about hospice, adult day care, home-care services, and advocacy programs in various countries. It is also possible to learn about Elderhostel programs, intergenerational programs, nursing homes, and respite care in every state in America and around the world. Technological access is an educational tool for aging persons in the new millennium.

References

American Society on Aging. 1999. *American Society on Aging Newsletter* (Nov.).

Australian Institute of Health and Welfare (AIHW). 1997. Aged and respite care in Australia: Extracts from recent publications. AIHW Cat.No. AGE.5 Canberra. AIHW.

Baumhover, Lorin A., and S. Colleen Beall. 1996. *Abuse, neglect, and exploitation of older persons: Strategies for assessment and intervention.* Baltimore, Md.: Health Professions Press.

Brashears, F., and M. Roberts. 1996. The black church as a resource for change. In *The black family: Strengths, self-help, and positive change,* edited by Sadye L. Logan. Boulder, Colo.: Westview.

Charging children for care of aging parents: Two Asian nations turn to family for cash. 1996. *Global Aging Report* 1 (4): 4.

Cohen, Gene D. 1997. Gaps and failures in attending to mental health and aging in long-term care. In *Depression in long term and residential care: Advances in research and treatment,* edited by R. L. Rubenstein and M. P. Lawton. New York: Springer Publishing.

Does the care suit the client? Reports on home help and a home-like environment. 1997. *Global Aging Report* 2 (6): 5.

Elderhostel: Adventures in lifelong learning. 1999. On-line: http://www.elderhostel.org

Geralnik, David, ed. 1974. *Webster's new world dictionary.* 2nd ed. New York: Williams Collins and World Publishing.

Harrison, James. 1997. Housing for the aging population of Singapore. *International Ageing Journal* 23 (3–4) (winter/spring): 32–48

Kara, Shabeen. 1997. Housing facilities in India. *International Ageing Journal* 23 (3–4) (winter/spring): 107–14.

Katan, Yoseph, and E. Werczberger. 1997. Housing for the elderly people in Israel. *International Ageing Journal* 23 (3–4) (winter/spring): 49–64.

Kim, Manjae. 1997. Housing policies for the elderly in Korea. *International Ageing Journal* 23 (3–4) (winter/spring): 78–89.

Kose, Satoshi. 1997. Housing elderly people in Japan. *International Ageing Journal* 23 (3–4) (winter/spring): 148–64.

Krout, J. 1998. Senior centers in America. In *Community resources for older adults: Programs and services in an era of change,* edited by R. Wacker, K. Roberto, and L. Piper. Thousand Oaks, Calif.: Pine Forge Press.

Lindstrom, Bente. 1997. Housing and service for the elderly in Denmark. *International Ageing Journal* 23 (3–4) (winter/spring): 115–32.

Saunders, Cecily, Dame. 1997. Hospices worldwide: A mission statement. In *Hospice care on the international scene,* edited by Dame Cecily Saunders and Robert Kastenbaum. New York: Springer Publishing 1999.

SeniorNet. 1999. On-line: http://www.seniornet.org

Shepherd's Centers of America. 2002. On-line: http://www.shepard.org

Stjernsward, Jan. 1997. The international hospice movement from the perspective of the World Health Organization. In *Hospice care on the international scene,* edited by Dame Cecily Saunders and Robert Kastenbaum. New York: Springer Publishing.

Tirrito, T., and J. Spencer-Amado. 2000. A study of older adults' willingness to use social services in places of worship. *Journal of Religious Gerontology* 11 (2): 35–42.

Wacker, R., K. Roberto, and L. Piper. 1998. *Community resources for older adults: Programs and services in an era of change.* Thousand Oaks, Calif.: Pine Forge Press.

Who are the likely victims? Reports on elder abuse. 1997. *Global Aging Report* 2 (5): 4.

Resources for the legal problems of older persons are:

National Senior Citizens Law Center. Washington, D.C.

American Bar Association, Commission on Legal Problems of the Elderly. Washington, D.C.

American Association for Retired Persons Legal Counsel for the Elderly. Washington, D.C.

National Center on Elder Abuse Washington, D.C. On-line: http:// www.elder-abuse.org

❖ Launch a campaign on healthy aging for all.
❖ Ensure that primary health care is accessible to the elderly.
❖ Provide support for the elderly so they may continue living in their own homes as long as possible or choose alternative accommodations.
❖ Provide and enhance accessibility and mobility for the elderly to jobs, social and health services, and leisure facilities.
❖ Provide key roles for older persons in voluntary or paid programs.
❖ Integrate the subject and activities of aging into national events. (Sen 1994, 126)

Impact on Business and Economy

The global economy will be influenced by new markets and businesses in leisure, educational materials, and technology catering to mature consumers. A concentration of wealth in the older population will increase their buying power and provide a market for services. The older population are a "comfort group." They seek products and services to ease age-related physical changes. They are financially able to buy clothes, toys, and gifts for grandchildren and to provide for their grandchildren's education and recreation. This cohort of older persons is physically active and will make every effort to maintain their physical stamina as long as possible by buying and using a variety of sports equipment, gyms, spas, health products, vitamins, herb supplements, etc. This longer-living group will need more clothes, food, leisure, and medicine for many more years than do previous cohorts.

In the United States, the Rand Center on Aging (a research and demography center) provides data about the aging population to the research community. The Rand Center reports on current research and policy issues in economics, demography, epidemiology, and health. Data currently available on the Contextual Data Library (web site: www.rand.org/centers/aging) are remaining life expectancy, Social Security average wage index, contribution rates for old age and survivor's insurance, disability insurance and hospital insurance, divorce rate and divorce law by state, and average poverty thresholds by family size (elderly and non-elderly).

These data inform the business community about the mature market developing in the United States, but the mature market is worldwide. In the United States, mature adults make up 75% of the travel market. "Age Power is creating a new mature market," writes Ken Dychtwald in his book, *Age Power: How the 21st Century Will Be Ruled by the New Old* (1999a). Seventy-six million Americans will be older than 50 years in the next decade. The 50 and older population represents a new age power. They control more than $7 trillion in wealth, or 70% of the total wealth. More than 79% of this group own their homes; represent 40 million credit-card holders; purchase 41% of all new cars; account for 51% of all over-the-counter drug purchases; and have the greatest net worth of any other age group (Dychtwald 1999a). In the United States, companies are testing upscale home-delivery services specializing in meals for those persons with conditions such as coronary heart disease, heart failure, and diabetes.

In Japan, a cosmetic company is developing products for a new group of consumers and uses older Japanese women in their advertising and marketing programs (*Global aging e-report* 1999). Also in Japan, older persons are encouraged to start business cooperatives with government support. The mature consumer will buy automobiles, houses, educational materials, technology equipment, leisure products, and comfort products. The buying power of older persons is evident in the long-lived older person who wants comfort products such as recliner chairs, easy-access automobiles, large-print reading materials, and safe environments. The older person is willing to try new products and new adventures. The media must change its image of the older person and show older adults using technologically advanced equipment, enjoying sports and sports equipment, traveling, and studying in new educational programs.

The demand for alternatives to nursing homes created a building boom in assisted-living facilities in the United States. Older people prefer home-like environments with medical supervision, and investors are realizing an average return of 17% annually (Better living through electronics 1996).

In Israel, the increase in the number of employed people with pension plans will contribute to better retirement living and to reduced dependency on government services and on their families. Growth is expected in private services. In Israel, there is a decline in the active labor force and increased numbers of retirees are participating in more leisure activities and community social involvement. The "new aged" of the future will seek new roles in community, employment, volunteering, and in educational facilities (Brodsky and Bergman 1993).

Impact on Health-Care Systems

Health-care systems probably can expect the greatest impact from the longevity explosion. Older adults will demand improved acute-care services; new pharmaceuticals; outcome-based mental health programs for depression, alcoholism, and anxiety; continuing-care communities in rural and urban areas; amenities in health-care environments; more research funding for age-related diseases; financial support for new technology such as laser eye surgery, plastic surgery, transplants, and orthopedics; improved dental and eye care; quality private and government home health-care programs; improvements in nursing home environments; easier access to respite care; access to hospice care; and more physicians, psychiatrists, and health professionals trained in geriatrics and gerontology. The senior market accounts for more than $610 billion per year in direct health-care spending, representing 65% of all hospital bed days and 42% of all physicians' office visits (Dychtwald 1999b).

Telemedicine (electronic house calls) offers health-care access to older Americans in rural areas. With high-speed cables, two-way television, and special projectors, this system links the medical personnel in urban hospitals with patients in remote areas (Better living through electronics 1996).

In Turin, Italy, the Institute of Gerontology began a Home Hospitalization Service to improve the effectiveness of health-care interventions for the elderly. Diagnosis and treatment take place in the home rather than in the hospital. A doctor-and-nurse team visits each patient at home to conduct an assessment of the home and the psychological and social functioning of the patient (Briefs: Retirement age 1994). Home-team visits will increase to provide more access to services, but the costs will also increase. Health-care systems may be challenged or burdened with financial difficulties because of these increased costs. A challenge to pharmaceutical companies is providing new products at affordable costs. Undoubtedly, pharmaceutical companies will benefit from the longevity explosion because the longer a person lives, the more drug products that person will likely consume.

The European Union increased its funding for Alzheimer's sufferers by 400% from 1993 to 1996. The European Union supports research on early diagnosis, methods of care, and support for families and care-givers (Services for seniors 1996). Long-term care costs can be expected to increase if the present state of disability in older persons continues. In Austria, anyone who needs long-term care for more than six months can apply for a long-term care allowance. The Austrian program is funded by a national social insurance program.

Every German is covered for the cost of nursing care in institutions or at home. Eligible persons may receive home-care benefits in cash, services, or a combination of the two. Financing is through a contribution of 1.7% of salary, with the cost split between employers and employees.

Israel provides long-term care insurance for all older Israelis living at home with home-care services. Family support is not a factor for eligibility. The program is funded by a contribution of employees' wages with contributions by the employer, employee, and the government.

Japan's long-term care insurance assists persons older than 65 who have physical and mental impairments. Coverage extends to in-home

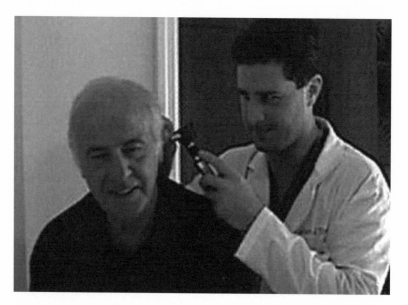

Doctors who treat older persons should be trained in geriatrics.

will be older and must prepare for its new members. Europe will be older, with a shrinking younger population to help support older persons. Africa must prepare for a new adult population. Aging persons can be a resource or a problem; which perspective is adopted will depend on the value placed on old people by their country. From the evidence in the literature, the ability to adopt strategies for aging populations requires recognition of the complexity of the lives of older persons. The appropriateness of strategies for each country will depend on the local context and the sociopolitical and economic factors of the country.

References

Aging everywhere. 1998. *Global Aging Report* 3–38. Washington, D.C.: AARP.

Better living through electronics: Innovations from Germany, South Africa, and the United States. 1996. *Global Aging Report* 1 (4) (Nov.): 5.

Briefs: Retirement age. 1994. *Aging International* 21 (4): 14.

Brodsky, J., and S. Bergman. 1993. Israel. In *Developments and research on aging: An international handbook,* by E. Palmore. Westport, Conn.: Greenwood Press.

Dychtwald, Ken. 1999a. *Age power: How the 21st century will be ruled by the new old.* New York: Tarcher/Putnam.

Dychtwald, Ken. 1999b. Age power is creating a new mature market. *Aging Today* 20 (6): 7.

Global aging e-report. 1999. On-line: http://www.aarp.org/intl/

Hsia, Lian Bo. 1993. China. In *Developments and research on aging: An international handbook,* by E. Palmore. Westport, Conn.: Greenwood Press.

Japan's Silver Human Resource Centers: "Life is studying and striving until you die." 1996. *Global Aging Report* 1 (4) (Nov.): 7.

Kaplan R., and E. Guglielmucci. 1993. Argentina. In *Developments and research on aging: An international handbook,* by E. Palmore. Westport, Conn.: Greenwood Press.

Kirk, Henning. 1993. Denmark. In *Developments and research on aging: An international handbook,* by E. Palmore. Westport, Conn.: Greenwood Press.

Kurtz, L. F. 1990. The self-help movement: Review of the past decade of research. *Social Work with Groups* 13: 101–15.

Long-term care elsewhere. 1999. *Global Aging Report* 4 (2) (Mar./Apr.): 2.

Powell, T. J. 1987. *Self-help organization and professional practice.* Silver Spring, Md.: National Association of Social Workers.

Sen, Kasturi. 1994. *Ageing: Debates on demographic transition and social policy.* London: Zed Books.

Services for seniors. European Union. 1996. *Global Aging Report* 1 (1) (May): 5.

Taking small steps toward security. Views from the Pacific Rim. 1996. *Global Aging Report* 1 (1) (May): 3.

U.S. Bureau of the Census, International Population Reports. 1992. *An Aging World II.* P25, 92–3. Data from U.S. Bureau of the Census, Center for International Research, International Data Base on Aging. Washington, D.C.: GPO.

CHAPTER TWELVE

Emerging Issues

In the new millennium a population of mature adults with diverse needs and strengths will change the world's view. Among the unresolved and controversial issues in Europe, Asia, Australia, Africa, North America, and South America are debates on extending life or improving quality of life, public policy choices or private choices, intergenerational conflict or interdependence, assisted suicide, the right to die, the role of spirituality and health, the search for technological medicine, and the identification of courageous agers. Predictions for the next millennium are based on the following assumptions:

❖ There will be many more older persons worldwide.

❖ We are keeping people alive into their seventies and eighties.

❖ Economic growth is generating increased personal wealth.

❖ Educational levels are increasing.

❖ We can expect an older population that is increasingly diverse—ethnically, politically, and economically.

❖ The economic status of older people will increase along with their purchasing power.

❖ We can expect a higher standard of living, even in retirement, due to the development of pensions, savings, health insurance, and support programs.

❖ Informal institutions are experiencing great stress in meeting human needs, from providing day care to feeding the hungry.

❖ Older adult volunteers can step in to take on the roles of previous stay-at-home mothers.

❖ Technology will be a powerful force, enabling older persons to remain productive by helping those who are disabled or ill to remain involved.

❖ Communications technology will bring us information about cross-national issues.

(Aging beyond the year 2000, 1997)

Longevity versus Quality of Life

The controversy over longevity versus quality of life can be summarized in this fashion: Should we strive to extend life or to improve the quality of life, and should resources be allocated to increase the number of years of life or the quality of life for older persons?

Technology improves quality of life with organ transplants, prosthetic devices, knee surgery, hip replacements, laser eye surgery, and other innovative techniques. Technology can extend life with intubations for comatose persons, transplants for persons with heart disease, and prosthetic devices or medical equipment to keep persons with Alzheimer's disease alive as long as possible. Governments spend astonishing amounts of money to keep alive patients who have minimal quality of life. Medical technology focuses on adding years to life rather than improving quality of life.

Public debates regarding setting limits to life and health care are controversial. Daniel Callahan, in *Setting Limits* (1987), *What Kind of Life?* (1990), and *The Troubled Dream of Life* (1993), argues that life-extending treatment should be limited by age. Callahan argues for a limit to health care for people who are 65 or older, or perhaps somewhere in their late seventies. He reminds us of the high cost of care and the inability of society to maintain increasing numbers of older persons at such high costs. He proposes that medicine should change its goals from extension of life to achieving a quality old age, and that developments in medicine should not focus on life-extending technologies such as organ transplants but should focus on comfort care for the last days of life (Schneewind 1994). An ethical dilemma for the twenty-first century will be how governments should spend their resources—on technology and research to extend life or on research and services that enhance quality of life.

Because preferences often are not made known before a crisis, physicians prefer to undertake certain treatments rather than have them withdrawn or not initiated (Smith 1996). Some physicians assess prognosis, cognitive deficits, limited life expectancy, and decreased quality of life when making treatment decisions, but to others extending life is the primary concern. Age-rationing of health care is an option.

In the United States, physicians are committed to extending life in spite of suffering and disability. Litigation and unclear legal guidelines create dilemmas for those physicians who would like to consider other options or the individual's preferences. Extreme levels of treatment are not the choice of between 73% and 85% of the adult population; additionally, about 86% of physicians would prefer no treatment for themselves (Smith 1996). However, fewer resources are available for quality-of-life studies than for scientific studies to extend life.

Public Policy Choices or Private Choices

Whether government or the individual should be responsible for health care, social services, and financial support is another controversy. Should government limit pensions and demand compulsory contributions by employees and employers? Who should make choices for older persons in the next century?

About twenty-five years ago, the living will document was designed to permit patients to have choices for end-of-life medical treatments such as intubations, gastric-tube feeding, suctioning, breathing machines, catheters, etc. Advanced directives and health-care proxy documents were legalized to permit individuals, rather than government, to choose from these options. In the United States, a person's right to die or to refuse medical treatment varies according to state law. In the Netherlands, the right to die is the individual's choice (Smith 1996).

Privatization of social security and compulsory savings plans are global controversies. Private plans are gaining in public support. In the United States, government is studying privatization of Social Security pension plans. Following the Chilean Model, in which private companies manage pension plans, the United States is considering private management of the Social Security pension. Globally, four basic sources of income for older persons are:

❖ Family support
❖ Personal savings
❖ Employer-sponsored pensions
❖ Public pension systems
   (Aging everywhere 1998)

In developing countries, family support is the foremost source of income. In the developed world, public and private pensions are widespread. Governments are cutting back pensions, raising retirement ages, limiting early retirement, and reducing benefits. Employees are asked to take more responsibility for their pension plans. Governments are encouraging, and sometimes enforcing, compulsory savings plans. Countries with mandatory savings plans include Malaysia, Singapore, and some African nations. Chile's pension system is managed by private companies (Aging everywhere 1998).

Globally, controversy exists regarding methods of providing financial security in old age. China instituted pensions for urban and rural dwellers. In Argentina, more than 90% of the population older than 75 years is covered by social security. With the increase in the aged population from 13% in 1987 to 16% in 2025, Argentina will be faced with a crisis (Kaplan and Guglielmucci 1993). Income support in Australia has been the government's responsibility since 1909; 85% of pensioners receive supplemental support from the government. Australia is experiencing a trend toward early retirement. At present, about half of all men between the ages of 60 and 65 are retired, and some states are considering legislation to prevent compulsory retirement (Lefroy 1993). China, Argentina, and Australia are among the many countries that must re-evaluate their pensions systems. Pensions systems, health-care choices, and other issues that affect the lives of the increasing numbers of older persons will be debated during the next century.

Intergenerational Conflict or Interdependence

Intergenerational conflict is inevitable if the younger generation is expected to financially and socially support the older generation. Rather, interdependence—an exchange of services among the young and the old—must prevail. The young and old should not compete for the same resources. Older adults contribute to the lives of younger persons by supporting pension systems, caring for young children, providing education to adolescents, and supporting the economic ventures of young adults. Older adults are able to contribute time and resources to younger persons. Young and old supporting each other will contribute to the well-being of both groups. The interaction between old and young without financial and social burdens (caregiving) must be a priority.

Japan and China provide examples of organized mutual exchanges between the young and old with employment programs. In Africa, the informal helpers of the old contribute to the economic success of the young. In other countries, older persons provide child care, volunteer to teach children and adolescents, and provide financial assistance to children and families who want to start businesses. Successful transition to an aging population demands interdependence rather than inter-generational conflict.

Ethical Dilemmas: Assisted Suicide/The Right to Die

The right to die and physician-assisted suicide are global controversies. Few countries, except the Netherlands, have a consensus that an individual has the right to choose when to die or if physicians should assist in the dying process. Prado (1990), a believer in individual choice, argues that suicide is sometimes the wisest course of action and discusses three types of suicide: surcease suicide; preemptive suicide; and suicide arising from despair, confusion, or compulsion. Surcease suicide is suicide committed by a terminally ill person who knows death is imminent within a short time and chooses to end the suffering. Preemptive suicide is suicide committed by a reflective aging individual who decides coolly and not under duress to die.

Should assisted suicide be an option for the terminally ill? Will legalization lead to abuses and the devaluation of persons no longer productive in society? The role of physicians in assisting the suicide of terminally ill patients is a topic of strong disagreement in the United States. The well-known Dr. Jack Kevorkian cases have tested the court systems. However, there is growing consensus that clinical protocols are needed to guide physicians in the process of assisting patients to die with dignity (Smith 1996).

Since the 1970s, the Netherlands has accepted the practice of voluntary euthanasia. In 1993, the Dutch Parliament became the first European country to officially permit euthanasia, but legislation did not legalize the act, which remains punishable by up to twelve years in prison. The Dutch government requires the physician to follow a detailed protocol if a person is permitted to die. The dilemma for societies is how to reach consensus in government or private choices (Smith 1996).

The Role of Spirituality/Religion

An issue for exploration and debate in this century is the role of spirituality and religion in research, treatment, and service delivery. The importance of religion and/or spirituality in the lives of older persons is well documented (Koenig 1997). Spirituality and religion reportedly influence health and mental health problems and treatments (Koenig 1997), but these questions need further exploration. Understanding the spiritual person is an unexplored area in health-services research and gerontology.

Gerontologists are studying the role of spirituality and religion and its impact on well-being, health, and longevity (Sapp 1996). Evidence is accumulating that religion positively influences health and psychological well-being (Koenig 1994)—in spite of the fact that researchers disagree on the operationalization of concepts of religiousness and spirituality. Koenig sees religion as the key to successful aging, writing, "Whether the religious perspective adds years to life has not been established, it is becoming more and more clear that it may add life to the years that remain" (1995a, 25).

Another issue of debate is whether medical technology has the ethical right to interfere with death. Are we playing God? Medical technology prolongs life using technology to assist eating, breathing, eliminating bodily wastes, and replacing organs that are no longer able to function. The case of Rita is an illustration.

> Rita, age 100 years, was a patient in a large teaching hospital in a big city. She was in a comatose state for nine months but was being maintained with a feeding tube, a breathing apparatus, a catheter for elimination, and was lying on a water-filled mattress to relieve the pressure of decubitus ulcers. She was well cared for by a staff of highly skilled nurses and physicians on a twenty-four-hour rotation. She was noncommunicative and nonresponsive. Rita had outlived her husband and children and did not have any relatives to make decisions for her. The hospital administration believed they were legally and ethically responsible to maintain her in this state as long as she lived. All known technologically advanced machines were used to keep death away.

Are we playing God?

The Search for Successful Aging

The search for a successful old age was of interest in the last century and most likely will be of interest in this century. Strawbridge suggests that "successful aging" is an American term. He writes, "It is a very American term, implying a kind of contest but there remains a search for paradigms of successful aging" (2000, 14). Nathanson and Tirrito (1999) believe that, in order to age successfully or live a successful old age, one must be a courageous ager.

Who is a courageous ager and how does one become a courageous ager? Nathanson and Tirrito (1999) define courageous agers as those persons who have focus, vision, and are willing to take risks. The journey to courageous aging is similar to climbing a mountain. A person must be prepared for the journey—physically, psychologically, and spiritually. Individuals must prepare in middle-age or early adulthood for the journey of aging if it is to be a successful achievement. The dimensions of courageous aging are psychological, biological, social, religious, and political. Assumptions of the model of courageous aging include these elements:

- Old age is a phase-in period from 60 to 70 years.
- It differs from individual to individual, based primarily on the health of that person.
- It assumes that aging is a different experience for every individual; some people are better prepared by endowment and/or life experience to manage the challenges of aging.

Losses occur at increased rates with the passage of years. Strength of character in old age is related to one's ability to overcome losses and cope with, or master, new challenges. Wisdom develops as the individual masters life's challenges and develops a greater ability to experience the richness of life. Nathanson and Tirrito (1999) describe the courageous ager as experiencing four pinnacle stages:

- Transience   (55–64)
- Early old age   (65–74)
- Middle old age   (75–84)
- Old-old age   (85 and older)

While the psychological and sociological (including financial and political) challenges of each pinnacle stage are different, the successful resolution of each pinnacle creates the potential for mastery of future challenges. The study by Nathanson and Tirrito (1999) explores the ability of the courageous ager to master and cope with particular challenges, including what factors promote and what factors impede an individual from experiencing a courageous aging resolution at the different phases of aging. What personality characteristics are exhibited by a courageous ager in managing various life challenges? The authors argue that social conditions impact the experiences of people as they age and promote or impede courageous aging opportunities. They ask, what can middle-aged people do to achieve their goals for aging successfully?

The material that evolved from the data indicated that a courageous ager is a *constantly evolving individual* who confronts different challenges at different life stages. In the early stage, *the complacency phase,* or middle age (ages 45 to 54 years), the individual should be deepening attachments and connections to the social world and developing a feeling of satisfaction (complacency versus dissatisfaction).

In the *transience phase* (ages 55 to 64 years), the major task is to begin to feel free from many of the social restraints of the earlier years and to search for new heights of experience. The task is to achieve *inspiration* or suffer the consequences of *apathy.*

In *early old age* (ages 65 to 74 years), the task is to develop *wisdom,* or the ability to transcend conventional thinking and develop one's own world view. Failure is associated with decline (wisdom development versus degeneration). In this stage, the mind takes precedence over factors related to physical functioning, and it is the spirit of the individual that helps prevail over difficulties.

In *middle old age* (ages 74–85 years), the e*ngagement phase,* there is a challenge to remain engaged in life in spite of the many changes in social roles and health status. Engagement versus detachment presents the challenge to find new ways of self-expression.

In *old-old age* (ages 85 years and older), the courageous agers are those who live in the present because they are able to make peace with the future. They remain in charge of their own lives and are in control even of their own dying. Courageous agers are those who believe that the future is shaped by today. The term, *courageous ager,* is more universal and can be applied with a global perspective to the older person of the next millennium. The search for "successful aging" is in the ability to be a courageous ager.

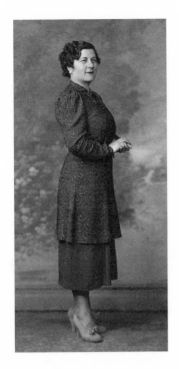

There are biopsychosocial differences in the 34-year-old woman of the 1930s and the 34-year-old woman in the new millennium.

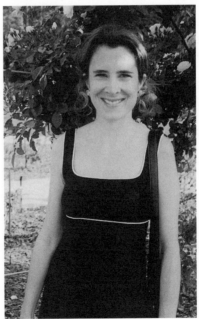

Summary

Aging in the twenty-first century will be very different from aging in the twentieth century. The older adult of the past will not resemble the older person of the future. Aging trends beyond the year 2000 will be historically unparalleled. The basic structures of societies will be re-examined and redefined to adapt to an aging population. Globally, controversies, debates, and ethical dilemmas must be resolved. The interdependence of young and old will be necessary to resolve these dilemmas and conflicts. It is hoped that a global society that is aging courageously will emerge from these controversies.

Poems

If I Had It to Do Over Again

In my next life
I will be able to
Eat all I want
And not gain weight
Play the guitar
And sing
Get a medical degree
And find the cure for cancer
Otherwise
I wouldn't change a thing

Natasha Josefowitz, Ph.D.

The Best Is Yet to Come

Don't have to climb
The corporate ladder
Don't have to be upwardly mobile
Don't have to move mountains
Or struggle with others
Don't have to set my sights
Upon some distant goal
Don't have to prove anything
Or cater to anyone
It's not uphill anymore

It's over that hill
With a lovely view
Of the best years
Yet to come

Natasha Josefowitz, Ph.D.

References

Aging beyond the year 2000. 1997. *Global Aging Report* 2 (4) (July/Aug.): 2.

Aging everywhere. 1998. *Global Aging Report.* Washington, D.C.: AARP.

Josefowitz, Natasha. 1995. *Too wise to want to be young again.* Boulder, Colo.: Blue Mountain Press

Kaplan, R., and E. Guglielmucci. 1993. Argentina. In *Developments and research on aging: An international handbook,* by E. Palmore. Westport, Conn.: Greenwood Press.

Koenig, H. 1994. *Aging and God: Spiritual pathways to mental health in mid-life and the later years.* New York: Haworth Press.

Koenig, H. 1995a. Religion and health in later life. In *Aging, spirituality, and religion: A handbook,* edited by Melvin A. Kimble, Susan H. McFadden, James W. Ellor, and James J. Seeber. Minneapolis, Minn.: Fortress Press.

Koenig, H. 1995b. *Research on religion and aging: An annotated bibliography.* Westport, Conn.: Greenwood Press.

Koenig, H. 1997. *Is religion good for your health? The effects of religion on physical and mental health.* New York: Haworth Press.

Lefroy, R. 1993. Australia. In *Developments and research on aging: An international handbook,* by E. Palmore. Westport, Conn.: Greenwood Press.

Nathanson, I., and T. Tirrito. 1999. Beyond the genome: An epidemiological view of successful aging. Paper presented at the Gerontological Society of America, November, San Francisco, California.

Prado, Carlos. 1990. *The last choice: Preemptive suicide in advanced age.* New York: Greenwood Press.

Sapp, Steven. 1996. Ethical perspectives. In *Aging, spirituality, and religion: A handbook,* edited by Melvin A. Kimble, Susan H. McFadden, James W. Ellor, and James J. Seeber. Minneapolis, Minn.: Fortress Press.

Schneewind, Elizabeth H. 1994. Of ageism, suicide, and limiting life. *Journal of Gerontological Social Work* 23 (1–2): 135–50. New York: Haworth Press.

Smith, George P., III. 1996. *Legal and healthcare ethics for the elderly.* Washington, D.C.: Taylor and Francis Pub.

Strawbridge, W. 2000. Chronic illness: Coping successfully for successful aging. *Aging Today* (Sept./Oct.).

This book began with a chapter on aging around the world, which covered life expectancy worldwide; the world's oldest countries; and the social and economic impact of global aging in Asia, Oceania, Europe, and South America. Aging in America focused on the old-old, baby boomers, and ethnic populations, as well as the social and economic characteristics of older Americans, with a report from a study of the concerns of older Americans.

The discussion of life expectancy presented statistics and research for developed and developing countries on life expectancy, as well as gender and ethnic differences in life expectancy. This discussion included theories of the causes of increased life expectancy, active life expectancy, and contrasting perspectives of implications of long life. With this basis, some factors that influence longevity were described, including genetics, personality, social class, and lifestyle considerations (diet, food restriction, vitamin consumption, exercise, and smoking).

Next, the physical and mental diseases that most commonly are found in older populations were briefly discussed and additional references were suggested for further study. Psychological factors, including attitudes about aging and myths about aging and the aged, are essential for understanding age-related behaviors. The diverse early experiences of women, ethnic minorities, and gay and lesbian older persons predict the future of these groups as they age.

Finally, personal and professional preparation is necessary to understand the impact of the longevity explosion on political systems, businesses, health-care systems, and social systems. Unresolved issues are the agenda for the next millennium.

Generalized Anxiety Disorder Self-Test

How much anxiety is too much? If you suspect that you might suffer from generalized anxiety disorder, complete the following self-test by clicking the "yes" or "no" boxes next to each question, print out the test and show the results to your health care professional.

How Can I Tell If It's GAD?

Yes or No? Are you troubled by:

❑ Yes ❑ No Excessive worry, occurring more days than not, for a least six months?

❑ Yes ❑ No Unreasonable worry about a number of events or activities, such as work or school and/or health?

❑ Yes ❑ No The inability to control the worry?

Are you bothered by a least three of the following?

❑ Yes ❑ No Restlessness, feeling keyed-up or on edge?

❑ Yes ❑ No Being easily tired?

❑ Yes ❑ No Problems concentrating?

❑ Yes ❑ No Irritability?

❑ Yes ❑ No Muscle tension?

❑ Yes ❑ No Trouble falling asleep or staying asleep, or restless and unsatisfying sleep?

❑ Yes ❑ No Does your anxiety interfere with your daily life?

Having more than one illness at the same time can make it difficult to diagnose and treat the different conditions. Illnesses that sometimes complicate anxiety disorders include depression and substance abuse. With this in mind, please take a minute to answer the following questions:

❑ Yes ❑ No Have you experienced changes in sleeping or eating habits?

More days than not, do you feel:

❑ Yes ❑ No Sad or depressed?

❑ Yes ❑ No Disinterested in life?

❑ Yes ❑ No Worthless or guilty?

During the last year, has the use of alcohol or drugs:

❑ Yes ❑ No Resulted in your failure to fulfill responsibilities with work, school, or family?

❑ Yes ❑ No Placed you in a dangerous situation, such as driving a car under the influence?

❑ Yes ❑ No Gotten you arrested?

❑ Yes ❑ No Continued despite causing problems for you and/or your loved ones?

Reference:

Diagnostic and Statistical Manual of Mental Disorders, Fourth Edition. Washington, DC, American Psychiatric Association, 1994.

If you or someone you know would like more information on generalized anxiety disorders, please go to the ADAA resource web page on this topic.

Reprinted with permission

Anxiety Disorders Association of America
8730 Georgia Avenue, Suite 600
Silver Spring, MD 20910, USA
Main # (240) 485-1001
Fax # (240) 485-1035

Source: http://www.adaa.org/AnxietyDisorderInfor/GAD.cfm

What's Your Bone IQ?

Do you know enough to prevent Osteoporosis?

Answer yes or no

❏ Yes ❏ No Do you believe that osteoporosis is a natural part of aging?

❏ Yes ❏ No Did you know that mild pressure like a hug can hurt an osteoporosis sufferer?

❏ Yes ❏ No Did you know that osteoporosis is essentially preventable?

❏ Yes ❏ No Did you know that osteoporosis can be stopped once it starts?

❏ Yes ❏ No Were you aware that over 70% of women with osteoporosis don't even know they have the disease?

❏ Yes ❏ No Are you aware that osteoporosis causes bone fractures for 1,500,000 Americans each year?

❏ Yes ❏ No Did you know that people who suffer from asthma, cancer, rheumatoid arthritis, thyroid irregularities and epilepsy are in a high risk group for osteoporosis? Medications used to treat these diseases promote bone loss.

❏ Yes ❏ No Did you know the amount of calcium needed for good bone health is the same for a 65 year old grandmother and her 14 year old grandchild?

❏ Yes ❏ No Did you know that osteoporosis is different from arthritis?

❏ Yes ❏ No   Were you aware that 10 years after menopause, a woman has lost 30% of her bone mass?

❏ Yes ❏ No   Did you know that one-half of those who suffer hip fractures never return to normal daily activities?

❏ Yes ❏ No   Did you know that exposure to sunshine or other sources of Vitamin D is necessary for your body to absorb calcium properly?

❏ Yes ❏ No   Are you aware that a bone mass density test is quick, painless and accurate—and the only way to know for sure if you have osteoporosis?

❏ Yes ❏ No   Did you know that osteoporosis has no obvious symptoms in its early state? That the first sign is usually an unexpected bone fracture?

❏ Yes ❏ No   Do you know how to assess your own risk for osteoporosis?

Check Your Score

How many times did you answer "yes"?

8–9 **Excellent Score**	No need to "Bone Up"
6–7 **Good Score**	You are very knowledgeable
4–5 **Fair Score**	You know some bone-saving basics
1–3 **Weak Score**	You need to "Bone Up"

Reprinted with permission

National Osteoporosis Foundation
1232 22nd Street N.W.
Washington, D.C. 20037-1292
Source: Web site: www.nof.org

GLOSSARY

Active life expectancy or **disability-free life expectancy**—The period of life that is free of limitations in the activities of daily living.

Activity theory—The theory that individuals will age successfully if they maintain their prior activity levels. Activity is the answer to finding happiness in old age; those who are not active are not happy.

Acute diseases—Temporary conditions or diseases such as infections or the common cold. These conditions decrease with age.

Age discrimination—A term that refers to discrimination on the basis of age.

Ageism—Refers to a negative attitude toward older persons.

Aging in place—Refers to those older persons who prefer to stay in communities where they have lived most of their lives.

Anxiety disorders—Refers to a constellation of symptoms. Some examples of these disorders are phobias, social phobias, agoraphobia, panic disorder, obsessive-compulsive disorder, and generalized anxiety disorder.

Apocrypha—An overall fragility that can lead to death in the absence of disease.

Attitudes—Manners of thinking, acting, or feeling that show one's disposition or opinions.

Baby boomers—A cohort of individuals who were born between 1946 and 1964.

Caloric restriction—Also called food restriction, or FR. It induces changes in cell membranes, delays the progression of immune deficiency with age, and protects and maintains cellular homeostasis.

Centenarians—A population of people 100 years and older.

Chronic diseases—Diseases that contribute to long-term health problems and dependency.

Cognition—The process of knowing in the broadest sense, including memory, perception, judgment, etc.

Compassionate stereotyping—Negativism describing older persons as persons who need help and persons who are disadvantaged at some level, either social, psychological, or economic.

Compression of morbidity—Older persons will experience a long, healthy, and active life with a short period of morbidity before death.

Congregate housing—A type of housing that includes apartments or houses for residents with shared facilities for meals and recreation.

Continuing-care retirement communities—Communities providing a full range of housing options from independent living to nursing home care.

Continuity theory—The theory that argues that the older individual will maintain the same or similar life activities or experiences that were experienced in early years in order to maintain stability.

Counter migration—A trend that refers to persons who return from the Sunbelt to be in areas with their family members.

Cross-linking—Concept that refers to the belief that an accumulation of cross-linked proteins damages cells and tissues.

Crystallized intelligence—Refers to the store of knowledge accumulated over time; is heavily influenced by education and socialization (vocabulary, associations, and technical skills).

Dementia—A syndrome with significant features such as impairment in short-term and long-term memory, impaired judgment, impairment in abstract thinking, and disturbances of cognitive functioning.

Dependency ratio—The number or proportion of individuals in the dependent segment of the population divided by the number or proportion of individuals in the working population.

Disengagement theory—A well-known aging theory stating that it is deemed necessary for individuals to withdraw from society to make room for younger persons in the society.

Double jeopardy—Concept that refers to being at risk from two disadvantaged social positions, i.e., being a woman and being old.

Ego differentiation—States that psychological adjustment is especially important at the time of retirement.

Endocrine theory—The theory that hormones control the pace of aging.

Epidemiology—The incidence and prevalence of common diseases.

Error catastrophe—Concept that refers to accumulating mistakes in the cell's ability to produce proteins.

Error theories—Suggest that environmental assaults to the human system gradually cause cells to malfunction.

Fluid intelligence—Describes performance or task, which is not influenced by level of education, such as response speed, attention span, and immediate reasoning ability.

Free radical theory—Speculates that oxygen radicals cause cells and organs to stop functioning and cause accumulated damage.

Gay gerontology—A field of study of older gay men and lesbians.

Generalized anxiety disorders—These disorders can be diagnosed when there are symptoms of excessive or unrealistic anxiety on most days for six months or longer.

Gerontology—A multidisciplinary field of study of the physiological and pathological phenomena associated with aging.

Gerontophobia—Fear of aging.

Global aging/worldwide aging—The revolutionary growth of aging in world populations.

Hayflick limit—The maximum numbers of divisions that normal human cells go through.

Health—A state of complete physical, mental, and social well-being.

Hospice—A philosophy of caring and an array of services for the terminally ill.

Immunological theory—The theory that a programmed decline in immune system function leads to increased vulnerability to infectious disease, aging, and death.

Life expectancy—The number of years, on average, that one can expect to live.

Maximum life span—The years that the human species has been documented to survive.

Medicaid—This U.S. program provides medical insurance for low-income families and individuals.

Medicare—U.S. program that provides national health insurance for older persons and is linked to Social Security payments.

Modernization theory—Describes the aging individual as being negatively impacted by modern society by having no role and being less valued.

Morbidity—An illness relating to or caused by diseases or days of sickness.

Mortality—The frequency of number of deaths in proportion to a population.

Normal aging—Changes that can be expected in most persons, i.e., wrinkling of the skin, graying of the hair, sensory or hearing changes, and changes in muscle tone, etc.

Nuclear family—Family usually composed of two parents and their children.

Obsessive-compulsive disorder—Disorder characterized by recurrent obsessions or compulsions sufficiently severe to cause marked distress or dysfunction in occupational or personal matters.

Old-old—The group of the elderly population, aged 85 years and older.

Panic disorders—Disorders manifested by somatic and cognitive symptoms such as palpitations, shortness of breath, chest pain, sweating, hot and cold flashes, fear of dying, fear of losing control, and fear of going insane.

Pathological aging—Refers to change or deterioration attributed to diseases as one ages.

Programmed senescence—Aging is a result of sequential switching on and off of certain genes, with senescence being defined as the time when age-associated deficits are manifested.

Random damage theory—Damage to mechanisms that synthesize proteins results in faulty proteins, which accumulate to a level that causes catastrophic damage to cells, tissues, and organs.

Rate-of-living theory—Argues that the greater an organism's rate of oxygen-basal metabolism, the shorter its life span.

Respite—Service that provides relief from caregiving responsibilities.

Sexuality—Refers to more than the biological functions of sexual intercourse and orgasm but also includes self-identity, expression of affection, intimacy, and pleasure in relationships.

Social exchange theory—The theory that a mutual exchange exists between older persons and younger persons in the form of support—emotional, financial, and instrumental.

Sociological theories of aging—These theories attempt to explain social phenomena in reference to their separate societal reality or, more broadly, an explanation system of social phenomena.

Somatic mutation theory—The theory that genetic mutations occur and accumulate with increasing age, causing cells to deteriorate and malfunction.

Stereotype—A fixed or conventional notion or conception of a person, group, or idea held by a number of people. This allows for no individuality or critical judgment.

Structural functionalism—Theory whose major concept is that "function" refers to the consequences of an action.

Successful aging—Refers to reaching old age with physical, psychological, and spiritual acceptance of this stage in life.

Symbolic interactionism—Explains how symbols are used for communication. A symbol is anything that gives meaning to a concept such as a flag, baptism, wedding, bar mitzvah, or funeral.

Triple jeopardy—Refers to having three risk factors such as being a woman, being old, and being a member of a minority group.

Wear-and-tear theories—Cells and tissues are said to wear out just as a car does after much use.

Work role preoccupation—Psychological concept in which self-worth is derived from work.

INDEX